RHEUM

RHEUMATOLOGY

A. K. CLARKE MRCP
Consultant in Rheumatology and Rehabilitation,
Royal National Hospital for Rheumatic Diseases,
Bath, UK.

Illustrations by Louise Allard

 CASTLE HOUSE PUBLICATIONS

First published in 1986 by
Castle House Publications Ltd
Castle House, 27 London Road
Tunbridge Wells, Kent

British Library Cataloguing in Publication data
  Clarke, Anthony
    Rheumatology.
    1. Rheumatism   2. Arthritis
    I. Title
    616.7'2   RC927
    ISBN 0-7194-0124-0

Typeset by M.C. Typeset, Chatham, Kent
Printed and bound by Billings and Sons Ltd, Worcester

CONTENTS

Acknowledgements

Tables 11.1, 12.1 and 12.2 have been reproduced from 'Rehabilitation in Rheumatology' (Clarke & Allard, 1986) by kind permission of Martin Dunitz, London.

CHAPTER 1

INTRODUCTION

This small book is intended to act as a simple reference book that can be carried in the pocket or kept in the case by the busy doctor who is seeing a range of rheumatological problems in his or her daily work – casualty, general practice, medical wards and in the orthopaedic department. The book is arranged in a regional fashion for ease of reference with sections at the end on arthritis in childhood and outlines of treatment. It is designed to be a working guide and hence there is a final section on further reading.

Scope of Rheumatological Problems

Arthritis and rheumatism are among the commonest afflictions of mankind. Rheumatoid arthritis has a prevalence of about 3 per cent in Western industrialised countries, which rises to 17 per cent in women aged over 75. Osteoarthritis occurs in anything up to 80 per cent of elderly people and back pain is one of the major causes of loss of production in industry. Indeed it is estimated that few people will escape a rheumatic condition in their lives. One in five consultations in general practice is for such conditions. However, the number of rheumatologists is relatively small and many other doctors are called upon to treat rheumatic patients. Arthritis frequently complicates systemic illnesses. Even more importantly most rheumatic conditions are treatable, and certainly the attitude that the patient must learn to live with the pain and immobility is totally unacceptable.

History and Examination

Rheumatology is essentially a clinical discipline; therefore the majority of diagnoses are made without relying on investigations, which are used mainly for confirmation or following the course of the disease.

An adequate history must be obtained. This is probably best done by taking a traditional medical history. The patient is asked to give his or her story in his or her own words. It is important to ensure that the story goes right back to the beginning of the problem as patients often refer to the present episode only, omitting previous episodes. This is particularly true in back pain. Patients also tend not to realise that pain in the feet has anything to do with a swollen knee, or that a stiff back is related to a painful shoulder. It is also important to ensure that when patients use a technical term that they are asked to explain what they mean by it. A good example is 'hip' pain, which usually turns out to be low back pain. Patients often repeat terms that other doctors, nurses, physiotherapists, etc. have used. This can be confusing and often wrong! A good example of this is the patient who is told he or she has cervical spondylosis or arthritis from the X-ray appearances alone, which are usually irrelevant and within normal limits for a patient of his or her age.

Once the patient has given the story, supplementary questions must be asked. With polyarthritis it is often worth asking about every joint that has not been previously mentioned to see if they have been affected, including the back. It is amazing how often the neck and back are not mentioned when they are involved, as many patients regard back pain as normal. If the patient has not specifically mentioned certain features these should be sought. Pain will nearly always be mentioned but swelling frequently is not, while stiffness is often missed out. Stiffness is a difficult symptom. If it is absent the patient is often mystified by the term, but if it is present the patient will readily admit to it even though the doctor and the patient may not be able to describe it in simple terms. Careful analysis shows that it is mainly pain. It is essential to ask about the time that the symptoms are worst. Inflammatory disease is worst in the morning or after prolonged sitting, while degenerative disease usually gets worse with activity, although there is often a short period of immobility stiffness first thing in the morning or after sitting.

With back or neck pain it is important to ask about paraesthesia, weakness and sphincter disturbance.

After the specific joint enquiry a much wider history must be obtained. This will include general questions about weight loss (or gain), fatigue and any other pre-existing medical or surgical conditions. Then a general health enquiry must be undertaken covering all the major systems, with specific enquiries about certain areas. These include skin rash, eye disease, urethral discharge and bloody diarrhoea. The past history occasionally gives an important clue. Much more rewarding often is the family history, which should include questions not only about arthritis, but about such conditions as psoriasis and ulcerative colitis. A social history is most important, especially where disability is present. Finally a drug history should be taken. This should include enquiry about previous analgesic, non-steroidal, second-line and steroid drugs.

The Examination

In a full rheumatological examination it is not enough just to look at the joint or joints complained of by the patient. It is essential to do a full medical examination, paying special attention to the skin, eyes, heart, lungs, abdomen and the nervous system. In the individual sections the special areas to examine will be highlighted.

When it comes to the joint examination a number of general points need to be made. As a rule all joints should be examined. The joint should be inspected, palpated and then put through its range of movement. Finally the function of the joint or group of joints should be assessed. The inspection should include looking for swelling, redness or other colour change, deformity and associated abnormalities such as muscle wasting. The palpation will reveal whether swelling is soft tissue, fluid or bony. Tenderness will be found and crepitus elicited on movement. The skin temperature will be determined. The patient should be asked to put the joint through its full range actively and then the examiner should find the full passive range. Any limitation of range should be attributed to pain or anatomical abnormality. Where appropriate the function should also be assessed. This is particularly important with the hand, shoulder, and lower limb when walking.

The individual joint ranges and important functional areas are given in Table 1.1. The examination of the joints is usually done badly and like examination of any other organ system, will only improve with practice. If the recording of the results of the examination is to be of value, then the actual measurements should be undertaken carefully using, if possible, a goniometer. It must be emphasised that there are considerable inter- and intra-observer errors involved in using such instruments, and again practice is required.

Interpretation of Investigations

Rheumatology is essentially a clinical subject. Investigations, including X-rays, will usually be used to confirm the clinical diagnosis and to assess the progress of treatment. It is pointless doing a battery of tests if the diagnosis is already made. False negative tests are frequently seen, and such investigations as rheumatoid factor and urate are fraught with difficulty if taken in isolation. In patients with widespread arthritis, especially in the presence of systemic disease, it is necessary to do a full haematological and biochemical screen. This is not just idle curiosity, but does allow a proper assessment of the overall effect of the disease process. Again the details of specific changes will be given in the individual sections.

If a specific test is undertaken it is important to be familiar with the normal values for the laboratory undertaking the test. Again it is emphasised that a positive test will only be of value in confirming a

Table 1.1 Range of movement of joints

Joint	Range (degrees)				Function
Cervical Spine	Flexion	45	Extension	45	Moving head
	Rotation	60	Lateral flexion	45	
Shoulder	(a) *with scapula fixed*				Hand placement
	Flexion	90	Abduction	90	
	(b) *with scapular movement*				
	Flexion	180	Abduction	90	
	Extension	50			
	Internal rotation	90	External rotation	90	
Elbow	Flexion	135			Bringing hand to mouth and rotation of forearm
Wrist	Extension	70	Flexion	90	Assisting hand function
	Radial deviation	20	Ulnar deviation	45	
Metacarpals	Flexion	90			Gripping and other skills
Proximal interphalangeals	Flexion	120			
Distal interphalangeals	Flexion	60			
Thumb	Should oppose ends of each finger				
Hip	Flexion	135	Extension	30	Standing, walking and sitting
	Abduction	50	Adduction	15	
	Internal rotation	45	External rotation	45	
Knee	Flexion	150			Standing, walking and sitting
Ankle	Dorsi-flexion	20	Plantar flexion	45	Walking
	Inversion	50	Eversion	10	
Toes	Dorsi-flexion	10	Plantar flexion	45	Walking

suspected or definite diagnosis. If a test result does not accord with the clinical state, question the test first, not the diagnosis.

When it comes to X-rays a number of points must be made. Firstly in many joint diseases the radiological appearences take time to develop. Secondly, global X-ray screens rarely give more information than carefully selected views. Thirdly, just because there is an abnormality on the X-ray it does not mean that it is that abnormality that is responsible for the symptoms. Lastly, X-rays are expensive and potentially harmful and thus should not be undertaken lightly. Again in the individual chapters the special X-ray requirements will be discussed.

Rheumatology is a subject which invades all areas of clinical medicine. As with all other branches of medicine, to be good at it, it is essential to practise the art and science of the speciality. Attention to detail, and especially taking a careful history as well as undertaking a meticulous examination, will usually enable a diagnosis to be made and a sensible course of treatment planned.

CHAPTER 2

POLYARTHRITIS

Definition

Polyarthritis is, as its name implies, any condition in which a number of joints are inflamed. By convention the number is in excess of four. The inflamed joints will be painful, stiff, swollen, warm and have reduced function. The term polyarthritis does not have any time implications.

Rheumatoid Arthritis

This is the classical form of polyarthritis. It is usually described as a disease of young women but can occur at any age from early teenage to extreme old age. Twice as many women as men get the condition but, because it is so common, it still occurs frequently in men.

Presentation

1 Seventy per cent of patients present as a small joint polyarthritis with prominent involvement

of the phalangeal–interphalangeal (PIP) joints, wrists and metatarsal–phalangeal (MTP) joints.

2 Twenty per cent present as large joint disease, involving the knees and shoulders as a rule. Often these patients have a more asymmetrical distribution of joint involvement.

3 Five per cent present with palendromic rheumatism. In this type there are sudden attacks of polyarthritis, with all the cardinal signs and symptoms of inflammation but only lasting a short time. This time ranges from 2 hours to 3 days and often will not be observed by the patient's doctor. The attacks come on at almost any interval. In the majority of cases the attacks come closer and closer together, and then become more typical rheumatoid arthritis.

4 Five per cent present with polymyalgia (see p. 94). The very prominent morning stiffness around the shoulders and hips may overshadow the arthropathy. As this presentation is most frequently seen in the elderly, it is an important diagnosis to make as steroids are not an appropriate method of treatment.

The frequency of joints involved in rheumatoid arthritis is shown in Figure 2.1.

5 Morning stiffness is common to all presentations. It may last a few minutes or all day. It is likely to be greatly modified by the use of analgesics, and careful enquiry should be made of the presence of stiffness prior to the use of the drugs.

6 Systemic effects are common. The most common are general malaise and fatigue. However nearly every system in the body can be

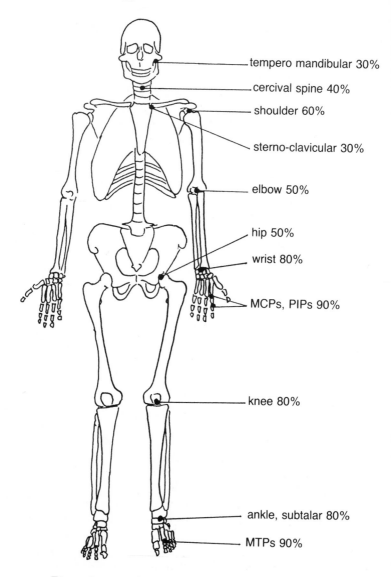

Figure 2.1   Joint involvement in rheumatoid arthritis

Table 2.1   Complications of rheumatoid arthritis

System	Complication
Cardiovascular	Pericarditis
	Valve lesions
	Myocardial granulomas
	Vasculitis
	Raynaud's phenomenon
Skin	Leg ulcers
	steroids
	vasculitis
	Felty's syndrome
Eyes	Scleritis
	Episcleritis
	Scleromalacia perforans
	Sjögren's syndrome
Lung	Fibrosing alveolitis
	Rheumatoid nodules
	Caplan's syndrome
	Pleural effusion
Neurological	Carpal tunnel syndrome
	Peripheral neuritis
	sensory
	motor
	mixed
	mononeuritis multiplex
	Spinal cord compression
Blood	Anaemia of chronic inflammation
	Bleeding from the gut
	Felty's syndrome
	Thrombocytosis
Soft tissue	Nodules
	Tendon rupture
	Ganglia
	Muscle wasting
	Tenosynovitis
	Bursitis
	Lax ligaments
	Amyloidosis

affected. These complications are listed in Table 2.1.

The physical findings in the joints will be given in the chapters dealing with individual regions of the body.

Some features should always be sought in rheumatoid arthritis, however:

1 Nodules. These occur over pressure points, most particularly the elbows and the dorsal surface of the forearm and in the Achilles tendon. They are also found in tendons in the hand and occasionally in the lung and eye.

2 Anaemia is frequent, giving pale mucous membranes and white nails.

3 Weight loss is evidence of active disease and the patient should be weighed at each visit.

4 Keratoconjunctivitis sicca is a common complication, especially in women, and dry eyes and mouth should be sought and specific tests (see below) undertaken if suspected.

5 Table 2.1 lists the systemic complications of the disease and if rheumatoid arthritis is suspected then all these complications should be excluded. This means looking for such signs as nail fold vasculitis, splenomegaly and fine crepitations in the lung fields, i.e. a full physical examination.

Investigations

Full blood count

(a) *Haemoglobin*. Anaemia is frequent. It is usually normochromic and normocytic. The evidence suggests that the anaemia is due to iron utilisation block and as such does not respond to iron therapy. However, many of the drugs used to treat arthritis cause blood loss from the gut and hence further investigation of the anaemia may be necessary. Figure 2.2 gives a flow diagram that can be followed under these circumstances.

(b) *White cell count.* This is usually normal but neutropenia is seen in the rare complication of Felty's syndrome which also features splenomegaly and evidence of frequent infections. Lymphopenia in the presence of arthritis should suggest systemic lupus erythematosus (see below).

(c) *Platelet count.* Active rheumatoid arthritis is usually accompanied by an elevated platelet count, sometimes to quite grossly high levels. As the arthritis improves with time or treatment the platelet level will fall.

Sedimentation rate and similar measures

(a) *Erythrocyte sedimentation rate (ESR).* This is almost invariably raised in rheumatoid arthritis. The ESR does not always accurately mirror disease activity.

(b) *Plasma viscosity.* This is an automated test which is favoured by some laboratories. Apart from giving an indication of disease activity it is specifically raised, to very high levels, in the rare complication of hyperviscosity syndrome which can lead to intravascular sludging and thrombosis.

(c) *C-reactive protein (CRP).* This is one of the acute-phase reactants. Many rheumatologists feel it is the best measure of disease activity. It is becoming widely available in many laboratories as a standard test. Other acute phase reactants, such as haptoglobin,

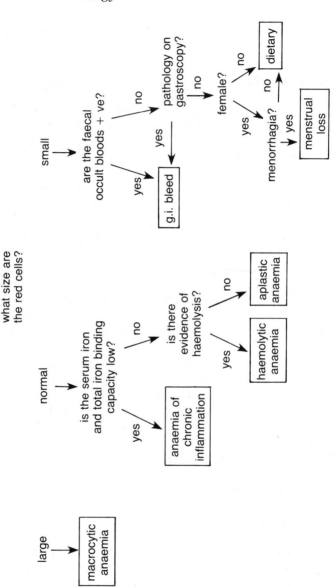

Figure 2.2 Flow diagram of anaemia in rheumatoid arthritis

alpha-1-antitrypsin and orosomucoid have no special advantages.

Biochemical tests

(a) *Urea*. The kidney is not usually involved in rheumatoid arthritis but a rising level might indicate the presence of amyloid in long-standing cases, although proteinuria should have been spotted first.

(b) *Liver function tests*. Although serious liver disease is not seen in rheumatoid arthritis, alkaline phosphatase acts as an acute-phase reactant and is frequently elevated. The fraction has been shown to be liver and not bone in origin.

(c) *Iron studies*. As mentioned above, the anaemia of rheumatoid arthritis is due to utilisation block. This means that the serum iron is often at very low levels but the iron-binding capacity is likely to be in the low normal range, meaning that there is not a lack of iron generally. Ferritin is the means by which iron is stored in tissues. Some is present in the blood and in patients without inflammatory disease a low ferritin level is the best evidence of iron deficiency. However, it acts as an acute-phase reactant and makes the interpretation of normal levels almost impossible, although low levels make iron deficiency anaemia almost certain.

Immunological tests

(a) *Rheumatoid factor*. One of the hallmarks of rheumatoid arthritis is the presence of the rheumatoid factor in the blood. This is usually a complex of IgM acting as an antigen with another IgM molecule acting as the antibody. High titres are common in active rheumatoid arthritis but it is not uncommon for positive tests to be found in normal people (5 per cent), elderly people (10 per cent), first-degree relatives of rheumatoid suffers (10 per cent) and in certain other diseases such as subacute bacterial endocarditis. The test therefore needs to be interpreted with caution. Several versions of the test exist. The simplest is the slide latex test which merely gives positive or negative. The tube latex and sheep cell test (Rose-Waller) are dilution tests and as such are a little crude in that there is the necessity for the laboratory to interpret the end-point of the reaction. More recently laser nepha-lometry has been introduced, which gives an absolute value for the amount of complexes present. Each laboratory will set levels at which the test will be regarded as positive.

(b) *Antinuclear factor (ANF)*. Although this test is associated with systemic lupus erythematosus it is positive in a wide range of disorders, including rheuma-toid arthritis. The test is a marker of tissue damage and if present in rheumatoid arthritis may herald serious complications, such as vasculitis.

(c) *Immunoglobulins*. These are frequently abnormal in rheumatoid arthritis but there is no consistent pattern that gives useful information in the treatment and diagnosis of the individual patient.

(d) *Tissue typing*. Although tissue typing is an im-mensely powerful research tool, at this time it has no place in the diagnosis of rheumatic disease.

X-rays

(a) *Plain X-rays*. Rheumatoid arthritis tends to affect

small joints. Therefore, for diagnostic purposes, X-rays of the hands and feet should always be performed. In the early stages soft tissue swelling and peri-articular osteoporosis will be seen. In the next stage erosions will appear. These occur at the margin of the synovial membrane (Figure 2.3) and on the ulnar styloid. It is wisest to avoid placing any significance on apparent erosions in the big toe metatarsal–phalangeal joint as this is frequently the site of trauma. As a rule, the distal interphalangeal joints will be spared. In the final stages there will be considerable disruption of the joints, with dislocation of the metatarsophalangeal joints, fusion of carpal bones, and destruction of major joints such as the knee and the hip. The range of joint involvement will be discussed in the chapters on the individual regions of the body.

(b) *Contrast X-rays*. The major use of contrast radiology in rheumatoid arthritis is looking for synovial fluid leakage following rupture of the knee joint (see Chapter 8).

(c) *Other imaging techniques*. The only one of much use in rheumatoid arthritis is the bone scan. This can be used in the early stages to show evidence of widespread synovitis which may not be obvious on clinical examination.

Biopsy

(a) *Synovial biopsy*. Samples taken blindly, at arthroscopy or at operation are very helpful if the typical appearances of the rheumatoid nodule are found (see Figure 2.4). However, this is unusual, and as a rule all one finds is a gross proliferation of the synovium with the infiltration of small round cells which the patholog-

erosions in the
metacarpals

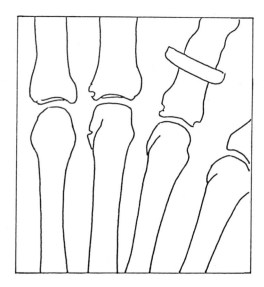

erosions in the
metatarsals

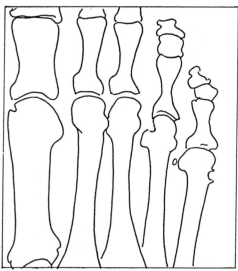

Figure 2.3 Site of erosions on X-ray

ist will usually report as compatible with rheumatoid arthritis. Such biopsies are most useful when they identify other, albeit rare, conditions such as tuberculosis.

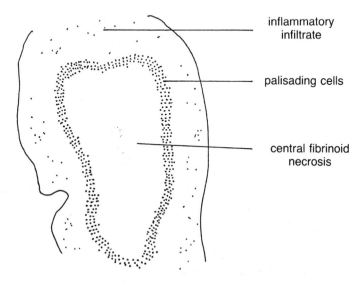

inflammatory infiltrate

palisading cells

central fibrinoid necrosis

Figure 2.4   The rheumatoid nodule

(b) *Nodules*. The highest biological correlate known in science is that between the rheumatoid nodule and the presence of a positive rheumatoid factor. In practical terms, if the rheumatoid factor is negative, then the lump on the elbow is not a nodule. Usually it is inadvisable to remove nodules, as they occur at pressure points. Healing may therefore be a major problem. However, a biopsy can make the diagnosis absolutely certain.

(c) *Fluid analysis*. The histological examination of

fluid removed from joints, together with culture, is used mainly to exclude other diagnoses, but the fluid removed from, say, the knee will be typically inflammatory in nature with large quantities of inflammatory cells, including neutrophils and also a wide range of small round cells. A typical cell has been described – the ragocyte, which is a large cell with a large number of intracellular inclusion bodies. The analysis of synovial fluid is discussed in more detail in Chapter 8.

Osteoarthritis (OA)

Although OA is often thought of as 'wear and tear' this is not so in the majority of patients. There is clear-cut evidence that the disease is, as a rule, a hereditary condition, more common in females than males. This form of the disease is called primary or generalised nodal OA. Secondary OA can occur in any joint that has suffered a previous insult, such as a fracture running through a joint surface, previous removal of a knee meniscus, or inflammatory arthritis, such as rheumatoid arthritis or gout.

Presentation

About half present with hand disease. The presence of Heberden's nodes, the bony cysts on the terminal interphalangeal joints, are pathognomonic of generalized OA (GNOA) and are described in more detail in Chapter 3. The interphalangeal joints can be involved (Bouchard's nodes) and when this happens there is the risk of the uninformed observer mistaking the condition for rheumatoid arthritis. The hands will be painful and stiff, although the morning stiffness tends to be much shorter-lived than that seen in rheumatoid arthritis. Frequently the involvement of the thumb base will make the hand painful on gripping. Women may present with fears about the appearance of the hands while both sexes may be worried that the hand disease foreshadows the onset of rheumatoid arthritis, especially if there is a family history of arthritis or rheumatism.

Other patients will present with involvement of one or more large joints becoming painful or functionally impaired. However, a careful examination of the hands will show the presence of Heberden's or Bouchard's nodes or involvement of the thumb base. The individual joints will be discussed in subsequent chapters.

Investigations

Laboratory tests

These are remarkable in OA by their normality. Unless there is intercurrent disease then the haematological and biochemical tests will be within the normal ranges.

X-rays

These are most helpful both with diagnosis and in deciding therapy, especially surgery. Typically there will be loss of joint space, due to the attrition of the cartilage, sclerosis and cyst formation, remodelling in the form of osteophytes and, in the end stage, gross joint destruction (Figure 2.5).

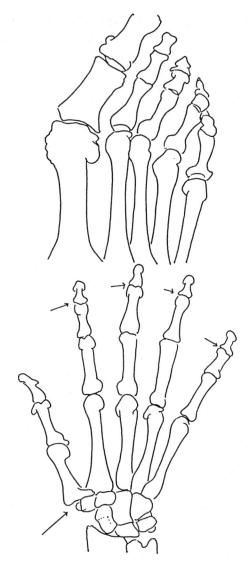

Figure 2.5   X-ray appearances of osteo-arthritis

Crystal Deposition Disease

Three types are commonly seen: gout, calcium pyrophosphate deposition disease (CPPD) and apatite deposition. Gout is the classical form of arthritis, being recognised from ancient times, but the other two have only been recognised in the past 20 years.

Gout

Presentation

This is the classical form of acute inflammatory arthritis. Typically it presents as a monarthritis affecting the big toe, knee, wrist or ankle. However it may present in a more polyarticular form from time to time, especially in well-established disease. In these patients there will be tophi present in the typical sites, the external pinnae of the ears, around the first metatarsal–phalangeal joint and adjacent to finger joints. Even in the chronic phase there are likely to be attacks of acute arthritis. These attacks are excruciatingly painful with considerable swelling, redness and loss of function. The skin overlying the involved joint, apart from being red, is tight and shiny and quite dry. Untreated the attack will last a week or so. Large joints such as the knee will often contain fluid. Removal of the fluid is not only important for diagnostic purposes but will also be pain-relieving. Tophi may well discharge the urate they contain in the untreated chronic disease.

Most gout is primary and related to hereditary

hyperuricaemia. Hippocrates was aware that gout was related to masculinity, stating in his Aphorisms that it was not seen in eunuchs, premenopausal women and prepubertal boys. This means that gout should not be entertained as a diagnosis in young women but must be remembered in the older woman. Primary gout is frequently precipitated by sudden changes in the biochemical status of the patient and is thus seen frequently after starting diuretic therapy, following major surgery or heart attack, during dehydration or fasting and following 'binge' eating or drinking.

Secondary gout is much less common but is seen when there has been an increase in purine metabolism as part of a disease, such as polycythaemia rubra vera, widespread secondary carcinoma or even extensive psoriasis.

Investigations

Biochemistry

(a) *Urate*. Gout is caused by the formation of sodium urate crystals in the tissues. Urate is relatively insoluble and it requires only minor changes in the physical environment of the body for these crystals to start to form if the serum urate is elevated. Hence this investigation is of the utmost importance in the diagnosis of gout. As with all tests it is important to be aware of the limits set by the individual laboratory but, as a rough guide, the normal range in men is 0.15–0.35 mmol/l(2.5–6.0 mg/100 ml) with women it is substantially lower, only rising to male levels well past the menopause. Hyperuricaemia can occur without clinical gout and therefore the result must be treated with care. Backache and a slightly elevated urate is not gout.

(b) *Blood urea.* In a small percentage of gout sufferers urate is laid down in the kidney, which in turn can lead to reduced renal function. Clearly this is a most serious complication; hence it is sensible to check that there is no elevation of the urea.

Examination for crystals

(a) *Synovial fluid.* The most certain way of making a diagnosis of gout is to identify urate crystals in the inflammatory joint fluid. If there is an effusion present in a joint, it should be removed for examination under the polarising light microscope. With normal light, the typical needle-shaped crystals will be seen occasionally within polymorphs which have ingested them. By using the polars the ability of the crystals to rotate the light, and hence appear brightly against the black background, will be demonstrated, and by the use of a first-order red filter the crystals will show strong negative birefringence (Figure 2.6).

(b) *Analysis of tophus.* Tophi sometimes discharge quantities of chalky material – monosodium urate. This can be examined under the polarising light microscope or, as there is much material available, can be chemically analysed.

(c) *Biopsy material.* Urate crystals can be identified in histological material, including specimens obtained at arthroscopy.

X-rays

(a) *Plain X-rays.* It is unsafe to base a diagnosis of gout on X-rays alone. Although it is true that the punched-out lesions around peripheral joints are fairly characteristic, if the clinical picture is so obscure that it

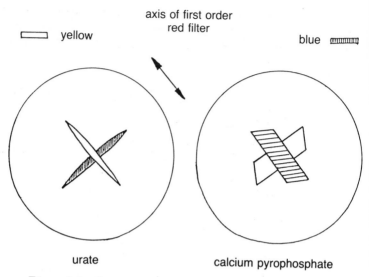

Figure 2.6   Crystals under the polarising light microscope

is necessary to resort to the X-rays, then the chances are that it is not gout.

(b) *Contrast X-rays.* Because of the risk of renal disease, intravenous pyelograms should be considered in any patient with long-standing gout with excessive tophi formation.

Calcium pyrophosphate deposition disease (CPPD)

Presentation

CPPD is due to the crystallisation of calcium pyrophosphate dihydrate in the tissues. This calcium salt is a normal intermediate metabolite in calcium metabolism. Why this should happen in certain people is uncertain. A very small number of cases are familial but the majority are spontaneous. The condition presents in two major ways. The first is as pseudogout in which there are acute attacks of monarthritis, usually in large joints such as the knee. These attacks are often recurrent and eventually lead to the degeneration of the affected joint or joints.

The second presentation is that of accelerated osteoarthritis. Practically any joint or group of joints can be affected, although the large joints are most commonly involved, especially the knees. Sometimes the amount of degeneration is considerable, with complete disruption of the joint.

Although the majority of cases are spontaneous, occasionally the condition is related to hypercalcaemia, particularly in primary hyperparathyroidism, haemochromatosis and hypophosphatasia.

Investigations

(a) *Biochemical tests*. In the spontaneous condition there are no abnormal biochemical (or haematological) tests. However, because there is the rare association with the disorders mentioned above it is essential to check the calcium, phosphate and alkaline phosphatase levels. The urine should be checked for glucose, and the blood for total iron-binding capacity and serum iron.

(b) *Fluid analysis*. The finding of CPPD crystals in synovial fluid confirms the diagnosis. These crystals are rhomboid in shape and are weakly positively birefringent on polarising light microscopy (Figure

2.6). These crystals may also be identified in histological specimens.

(c) *X-rays*. CPPD shows up as discrete cartilaginous calcification. Ninety-five per cent of sufferers will have evidence of calcification in the knees, both in the menisci and the hyaline cartilage (Figure 2.7). Other common sites of calcification are the symphysis pubis, triangular ligament in the wrist, the shoulder and the hip.

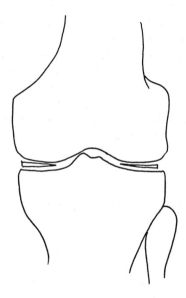

Figure 2.7   Meniscal calcification in pyrophosphate arthropathy

Apatite deposition disease

Hydroxyapatite is another intermediate metabolite of calcium. The crystals are very much smaller than those of urate or CPPD. The crystals are found in tendons and bursae and are clinically most important in the painful arc syndrome in the shoulder (see Chapter 4). It has been suggested that apatite may be responsible for some, if not all, cases of osteoarthritis.

Connective Tissue Disease

The diseases in this group affect a small number of patients but are distinctive and potentially serious. It is beyond the scope of this book to describe at length all the separate syndromes that occur, especially as a large number of overlap syndromes are now described. Rather the features that should raise suspicions of the diseases, together with the basic interpretation of the investigations commonly undertaken, will be discussed. Further reading suggestions are given at the end of the book.

Systemic lupus erythematosus (SLE)

Presentation

It is now recognised that this condition is much more common than previously thought, generally more benign and affecting a wider population. SLE can present in many different ways and should appear in most differential diagnoses for systemic disease. Table 2.2 gives the major complications and associations of SLE.

Table 2.2   Complications of systemic lupus erythematosus

System	Complication
Musculoskeletal	Arthralgia
	Synovitis
	Non-erosive arthritis
	(rarely: erosive arthritis, Jaccoud's arthritis)
	Aseptic necrosis
	Tendonitis
	Myositis
	Myasthenia
Skin	Butterfly rash
	Photosensitivity
	Chronic discoid lesions
	Alopecia – both scarring and non-scarring
	Petechiae, purpura and ecchymoses
	Non-specific maculopapular lesions
	Raynaud's phenomenon
	Diffuse hyperpigmentation
	Urticaria
	Leg ulcers
	Thrombophlebitis
	Livedo reticularis
Nervous system	See Table 2.3
Renal	Focal glomerulonephritis
	Diffuse proliferative glomerulonephritis
	Membranous glomerulonephritis
	Mesangial lupus nephritis
	Renal tubular acidosis
	Renal vein thrombosis
Pulmonary	Pleurisy
	Pleural effusion
	'Shrinking lungs'
	Pulmonary fibrosis
Cardiovascular	Pericarditis
	Cardiomyopathy
	Libman–Sachs endocarditis
	Vasculitis
	Raynaud's phenomenon
	Thrombophlebitis
Blood	Normochromic normocytic anaemia
	Haemolytic anaemia
	Leucopenia

Table 2.2 (cont.) Complications of systemic lupus erythematosus

System	Complication
Blood (cont.)	Lymphopenia
	Thrombocytopenia
	Clotting defects
Pregnancy	Spontaneous abortion
	Congenital heart block

(a) *Arthritis*. Virtually all cases will complain of joint symptoms at some time. Often this takes the form of arthralgia alone. This can be very severe and may be dismissed in the absence of florid synovitis. When there is actual arthritis the amount of synovitis is likely to be limited and it is most unusual for deformity to occur, with the exception of swan-necking (see Chapter 3).

(b) *Skin*. The classical skin lesion is the facial butterfly rash (Figure 2.8). However a wide range of fairly

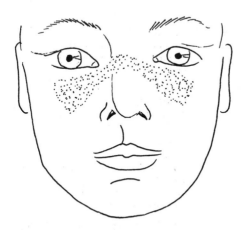

Figure 2.8 Distribution of facial rash in systemic lupus erythematosus

non-specific rashes may be seen, although there is a marked tendency for such rashes to be light-sensitive and for the disease in general to be worse after exposure to sunlight. Hair loss is common and SLE is one of the causes of scarring alopecia.

(c) *Renal*. One of the most serious complications of SLE is glomerulonephritis. Three types are described: focal, diffuse proliferative, and membranous. Focal is the most common but also the most benign. Diffuse proliferative is the most serious while membranous is the least common, again with a fairly good prognosis. Renal disease presents in a number of ways. Firstly it may be identified by the vigilant doctor carefully following a patient with known SLE. It may present with nephrotic syndrome (especially the membranous lesion), haematuria, acute renal failure or with hypertension. It is wise to routinely examine the urine of SLE patients.

(d) *Neurological*. The other serious complications of SLE are the neuropsychiatric ones, most notably psychosis and hemiplegia. Table 2.3 lists the principal neurological lesions seen. Any patient with SLE who develops a psychiatric or neurological lesion should be carefully screened for worsening disease, and any patient with an unexpected or unusual neurological condition should be investigated for SLE.

Table 2.3 *Neurological complications of systemic lupus erythematosus*

Depression	Cranial nerve palsies
Psychosis	Peripheral neuropathy
Epilepsy	Ataxia and chorea
Hemiplegia	Retinopathy
Paraplegia	

Investigations

Full blood count

(a) *Haemoglobin*. There may well be an anaemia of chronic inflammation with a normochromic, normocytic picture. SLE is also one of the causes of haemolytic anaemia and a Coombs' test is always worthwhile.

(b) *White cell count*. Although the total count is likely to be normal, a relative lymphopenia is common and has been regarded as diagnostic by some authors.

(c) *Platelets*. Thrombocytopenia, albeit mild, is common. There is overlap with idiopathic thrombocytopenic purpura and both are related to the production of antiplatelet antibodies.

(d) *Sedimentation rate*. SLE is one of the causes of ESRs in excess of 100. It is most unusual to see an untreated patient with the condition without a grossly elevated ESR, and even in patients apparently in clinical remission the levels are still likely to be high. By the same token other measures of 'unwellness', such as the plasma viscosity and the c-reactive protein, will also be elevated.

Biochemical tests

(a) *Urea and electrolytes*. Because renal disease is such a worrying complication of SLE, this is an essential test to repeat at regular intervals. A steadily rising urea may be the first indication of trouble.

(b) *Liver function tests*. Liver disease is extremely rare in SLE but it is not unusual for there to be a mild elevation of the alkaline phosphatase.

Immunological tests

(a) *Antinuclear antibodies (ANA)*. Previously known as the antinuclear factor, these autoantibodies are the hallmark of the disease. As mentioned above, they are not specific and can occur in a wide range of diseases where there is tissue breakdown, but they are seen almost invariably in SLE and in high titres. With the demise of the LE cell test (which was time-consuming and inaccurate if not done with great care) the ANA is now regarded as the screening test for SLE. Although it is possible to see SLE without a positive ANA this is very much a specialist diagnosis. The ANA is performed by indirect immunofluorescence, using a substrate such as rat liver. Different staining patterns are seen, including homogeneous, peripheral, speckled and nucleolar. The peripheral pattern correlates with the presence of significant anti-DNA antibody titres (see below) and hence the pattern most seen in 'true' SLE.

(b) *DNA antibodies*. Much more specific than the ANA is the presence of anti-DNA antibodies. The most frequent test undertaken in the average laboratory is the so-called DNA-binding test, which is not only highly specific for SLE but can be used to follow the course of the disease.

(c) *Complement studies*. Complement is a group of globulins which react in a cascade fashion like that seen in blood coagulation and which are essential in many immunological reactions. The formation of antibody–antigen complexes leads to the consumption of complement, especially the C4 component, and this can be used to follow the course of the disease, particularly the renal involvement.

(d) *Other immunological tests*. Space precludes a discussion of the whole range of immunological abnormalities seen in SLE and the related diseases, other than those mentioned briefly in the sections below. Suffice it to say that it is common to find antibodies present to a wide range of body constituents in the blood.

Urinalysis

As mentioned above, it is sensible to test the urine regularly to look for microscopic haematuria, albuminuria, and the presence of casts, which can all herald renal disease.

X-rays

(a) *Plain X-rays*. These are of use firstly in differentiating the disease from rheumatoid arthritis. Despite the considerable arthralgia there is rarely any evidence of erosive changes in SLE, so if these are present then the disease is likely to be rheumatoid arthritis. Secondly, plain films of the chest can be used to identify pleural effusion, pulmonary infiltrates and pericarditis.

(b) *Contrast X-rays*. In the presence of suspected renal disease an intravenous pyelogram is a useful investigation. Apart from excluding other renal lesions, it is necessary to identify accurately the location of the kidneys if a renal biopsy is contemplated.

Arteriography may be needed to identify vasculitic lesions in various sites such as in cerebral disease or in an acute abdominal crisis in a patient with active vasculitis.

(c) *Other imaging techniques*. CT scans and radioactive oxygen scans may be of use in cerebral disease, especially to differentiate intercurrent disease.

Biopsy

(a) *Skin*. The so-called lupus band test identifies the presence of deposits of gammaglobulin, usually in the dermal–epidermal junction. A positive test is highly specific for SLE, being seen in 90 per cent of affected SLE skin and at least 50 per cent of samples of apparently normal skin in SLE sufferers.

(b) *Renal biopsy*. As stated above, there is a range of glomerulonephritic lesions seen and, as they have different prognostic significance, a renal biopsy is usually necessary. The specimen will need to be examined under both the light and the electron microscope.

Scleroderma

This rare group of conditions may well present with joint pain, and needs to be considered in the differential diagnosis of any unusual arthropathy.

Presentation

(a) *CRST syndrome*. This is the benign form of the disease. The initials stand for calcinosis, Raynaud's phenomenon, sclerodactyly, and telangiectasia. The calcinosis is usually seen in the finger-ends on X-ray, but on occasion may be seen under the skin or even be extruded through digital ulcers. The Raynaud's phenomenon is among the severest seen, and autoamputation of gangrenous fingertips is a constant worry, especially in winter weather. The term sclerodactyly refers to the thickening of the skin, with the tethering down of the subcutaneous structures. The skin has a peculiar woody feel and as the condition progresses the fingers become increasingly flexed and non-functional. Tightness of the skin is also seen around the mouth, which becomes obviously smaller with the passage of time and the face may become expressionless due to the loss of facial wrinkles. It is often helpful to ask the patient to bring an old photograph along to the clinic to identify these facial changes. Examination of the face will also reveal the telangiectasia, which are likely also to be visible on the hands. The oesophagus is frequently involved in the CRST syndrome, with lack of motility, leading to dysphagia. The CRST syndrome has an extended course and is usually insidious in its onset.

(b) *Progressive systemic sclerosis (PSS)*. This condition is at the other end of the spectrum to the benign CRST syndrome. There is multi-system involvement, with death often occurring in a relatively short time due to renal or cardiac involvement. The typical skin changes are likely to occur but, because of the rapidity of progression in some cases, the more longstanding features, such as calcinosis, may well never develop. The whole gut is likely to become thickened and malabsorption is a serious problem. Sjögren's syndrome is a constant feature. Fibrosing alveolitis is frequent and can be disabling, while myocardial fibrosis and conduction defects can cause shortness of breath, as well as being life-threatening. Renal disease is manifest by hypertension and is a poor prognostic feature. A quarter of the patients get a small joint polyarthritis. A full list of the features of PSS is given in Table 2.4. It must be emphasised that there is a spectrum of scleroderma with PSS at one end and CRST at the other. Many cases of scleroderma have a combination of cutaneous and visceral disease.

Table 2.4 *Features of progressive systemic sclerosis*

System	Complication
Skin	Raynaud's phenomenon
	Thickening
	Tightening
	Loss of skin appendages
	Telangiectasia
	Calcinosis
	Increased capillary loops
	Ulceration
	Sclerodactyly
	Pigmentation
	Vitiligo
Gut	Sjögren's syndrome
	Microstomia
	Loss of oesophageal motility
	Malabsorption
Lung	Fibrosing alveolitis
	Massive fibrosis
	Reflex pneumonitis
	Pulmonary hypertension
	Alveolar-cell carcinoma
Heart	Myocardial fibrosis
	Conduction defects
	Fibrotic pericarditis
Kidney	Malignant hypertension
Muscle	Myopathy
Joints	Arthralgia
	Polyarthritis

(c) *Other scleroderma syndromes.* Localised scleroderma and a number of related conditions are described. They are all rare and are briefly described in Table 2.5.

Investigations

Full blood count

(a) *Haemoglobin.* There may be a mild normocytic,

Table 2.5   Rare scleroderma syndromes

Localised scleroderma		
(a)	Morphea	Localized patches of scleroderma, with no systemic involvement
(b)	Linear scleroderma	Linear streaks, including coup de sabre; binding down of underlying muscles
Eosinophilic fasciitis		Symmetrical and widespread inflammation of the deep fascia, subcutis and dermis, with marked eosinophilia
Vinylchloride disease		Acro-osteolysis associated with industrial exposure

normochromic anaemia (the anaemia of chronic inflammation). Rarely a haemolytic anaemia is seen. When there is extensive gut involvement there is likely to be iron deficiency anaemia or even macrocytosis.

(b) *Platelets*. Thrombocytopenia has been described.

(c) *Sedimentation rate*. The ESR is frequently normal or only just elevated, and therefore of little value in scleroderma, either in aiding diagnosis or following the course of the disease.

Biochemical tests

(a) *Urea and electrolytes*. Because renal disease is important, a watch should be kept on the urea and electrolytes.

(b) *Liver function tests*. Although hepatic involvement in scleroderma is virtually unknown, there is a well-described association with primary biliary cirrhosis. An elevated alkaline phosphatase should therefore alert the doctor to this possibility.

Immunological tests

(a) *Antinuclear antibodies (ANA)*. These are frequently found in scleroderma. The pattern normally observed is either the nucleolar or the speckled pattern, the latter being seen more in overlap syndromes.

(b) *Anti-centromere antibodies*. This antibody is fairly specific for scleroderma and, although at the moment it is mainly a research tool, it may well become more widely available.

X-rays

(a) *Plain X-rays*. Plain films of the hands may well reveal subcutaneous calcinosis and the absorption of the ends of the distal phalanges (acrolysis) which accompanies advanced disease. Plain chest X-rays will reveal 'honeycomb' lung and diffuse fibrosis.

(b) *Contrast X-rays*. In suspected scleroderma a barium swallow will confirm the lack of motility so typical of the disease, while small bowel studies may show dilatation and a barium enema may show dilatation and rigidity.

Biopsy

(a) *Skin*. Typically the skin will show hypertrophy of collagen with a marked paucity of skin appendages, such as sweat glands and hair follicles.

(b) *Renal*. In patients with kidney involvement the appearances are those of severe hypertension, with fibrinoid changes in arterial walls.

Dermatomyositis and polymyositis

These two conditions are closely related, the only

difference between the two being the presence of skin lesions in dermatomyositis. Two distinct varieties occur: childhood and adult disease. The differences between the two age groups are three-fold. In children the disease is self-limiting and is associated with marked subcutaneous calcification in a proportion of cases. In adults there is probably an increased incidence of malignant disease, although this is disputed.

Presentation

Muscle

Proximal weakness is the hallmark of the disease. Patients will report that they are having difficulty raising their arms, and that walking is becoming difficult. This weakness is made worse by fatigue. As the disease progresses there will be increasing difficulty with trunk and head control and eventually respiration. Examination will reveal good strength in the hands and feet but if proximal strength is examined marked weakness will be present. The best way of demonstrating this is to ask the patient to lie flat. The patient is then asked to fold the arms across the chest and then try to sit up. Most people can achieve this without difficulty, if the examiner holds the legs down on the couch. The myositis patient will have extreme difficulty, however. If proximal limb muscles are palpated in active myositis they will be tender.

Skin

There are a wide range of rashes to be observed in dermatomyositis. Even in polymyositis, one physical sign is commonly seen and that is dilatation of the capillary loops in the nail beds of the fingers. The other two classical skin lesions in dermatomyositis are so-called collodion patches on the knuckles which are raised and a little scaly, and, the classical purple (or heliotrope) rash seen on the face and especially the eyelids. A wide range of non-specific rashes may be seen on the trunk and limbs.

Joints

About a third of patients develop a small joint polyarthritis, mainly in the fingers.

Investigations

Full blood count

(a) *Haemoglobin.* As with most other chronic inflammatory diseases there is likely to be a normochromic, normocytic anaemia which will not respond to iron treatment.

(b) *Sedimentation rate.* The ESR in myositis is almost invariably raised. This also applies to other measures of 'unwellness' such as plasma viscosity and C-reactive protein.

Biochemical tests

Creatinine phosphokinase (CPK) is found in the circulating blood in small quantities but if there is muscle breakdown, as occurs in myositis, then high levels will be found. The CPK is nearly always raised in myositis and can be used as a very sensitive marker of disease progress.

X-ray

There are no specific X-ray appearances in myositis,

with the exception of the subcutaneous calcinosis of the childhood disease. However in adults it is expedient to make a search for a possible underlying malignancy and most authorities would agree that a minimum of chest X-ray, barium meal and enema, and intravenous pyelogram is needed.

Electromyography (EMG)

Probably no other disease relies so much on EMG for diagnosis. The typical findings of fibrillation at rest with bursts of polyphasic units are shown in Figure 2.9.

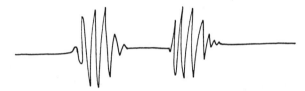

Figure 2.9   Polyphasic units on E.M.G. in polymyositis

Biopsy

Muscle biopsy is again a crucial investigation in dermatomyositis or polymyositis. Typically the biopsy will show a variable degeneration of individual muscle fibres with a widespread infiltration of small round cells. In the later stages there will be fibrosis with marked muscle atrophy. Prior to undertaking the procedure, it is important to discuss with the pathologist the method of acquiring the muscle biopsy. This is because damage to the specimen is likely to occur unless it is handled properly and the laboratory is expecting the specimen. Great care must be taken to avoid muscles that have previously been the site of EMGs as the needling can produce inflammatory changes that are difficult to differentiate from active myositis. Most units undertaking a lot of investigation of possible myositis will confine biopsy to the muscles on the right-hand side of the body, with EMGs being performed on the left.

Mixed connective tissue disease (MCTD)

Overlap syndromes are common (relatively) with the connective tissue diseases and it is often difficult to be absolutely certain what illness is being looked at. The best worked-out of the overlap syndromes is MCTD. It was first identified by the discovery of a specific antibody, that against extractable nuclear antigen (ENA). When patients, with what was thought to be SLE, were tested for ENA they were found to fit into a specific disease pattern. They had features of polymyositis, with muscle weakness, scleroderma, typical skin changes, SLE, arthralgia and photosensitive rash. It was found that these patients had a good prognosis and clearly formed a subset of SLE. It is beyond the scope of this book to discuss this topic further but readers should be aware of the possibility of overlap in connective tissue disease.

Seronegative Arthritis

As the classification of the rheumatic diseases improved after the Second World War, it became clear that there was a group of fairly common arthritic conditions that were different from rheumatoid arthritis because there was the absence of the rheumatoid factor. More careful analysis showed that inflammation of the spine was common. It was not until the early 1970s that it was found that there was a strong genetic link, the presence of the HLA-B27 antigen, that marked this group of diseases out as a discrete group with much to tell medicine about the aetiology of many chronic diseases. Ankylosing spondylitis is the classic condition of the group.

Ankylosing spondylitis (AS)

Presentation

Back pain

AS is essentially a form of arthritis of the spine. As such, the hallmarks of the disease are back pain with marked morning stiffness. The differentiation from other forms of back pain is discussed in Chapter 6.

Peripheral arthritis

In many patients with AS there will be arthritis in joints other than those in the spine. Hip disease is very common and these joints are only spared in the mildest of disease. Some authorities have even suggested that the hips should be regarded as spinal joints because of their frequent involvement in AS. Similarly the shoulders are often involved. Other peripheral joints are much less commonly affected but from time to time a patient is seen with a widespread polyarthritis. It is often stated that AS is predominantly a disease of young men but it has become clear, with careful epidemiological study, that it is as common in women but that it tends to be much milder, and it is often atypical when it is seen. Thus back pain may be much less of a feature than an inflammatory arthritis affecting the knees or similar joints.

Systemic complications

(a) *The eye*. Acute anterior uveitis (iridocyclitis) is common and can be disabling. The condition is usually unilateral with severe pain in the globe with obvious inflammation. A close examination of the eye will reveal injection of the blood vessels of the white of the eye and sometimes pus in the anterior chamber itself. The pupil may well be irregular due to the adherence of the iris to surrounding structures. If a strong light is shone in the contralateral eye, pain will result in the affected eye because of the consensual reaction. Examination of the back of the cornea in the apparently normal eye may well reveal little dark specks which represent precipitates due to previous anterior uveitis.

(b) *The heart*. The aortic valve may become inflamed in AS; hence the heart should be carefully auscultated to exclude the early diastolic murmur of aortic incompetence. This is best done with the patient sitting forward, with the breath held in expiration and the diaphragm of the stethoscope held at the left sternal edge in the second interspace or at the lower end of the sternum.

Investigations

Full blood count

(a) *Haemoglobin*. As with other inflammatory arthropathies there may well be a normochromic, normocytic anaemia. However, it is likely to be much milder than that seen with, say, rheumatoid arthritis.

(b) *Sedimentation rate*. The ESR is a disappointing investigation in AS. Quite often it is in the normal range and an ESR of 10 cannot be taken as evidence against active spondylitis. In fact none of the non-specific tests is of much use in following the disease.

Immunological tests

By definition AS is seronegative, which means that the latex test and the other measures of rheumatoid factor will be negative.

X-rays

(a) *Pelvis*. The most constant radiological feature of AS is sacroilitis. It is unsafe to make a diagnosis of AS if the sacroiliac joints are normal. The first change seen is a widening of the joint with erosive change and surrounding sclerosis. The joint then begins to obliterate and finally may totally fuse. It should be noted that it is very difficult to observe the early changes in the adolescent joint as the young pelvis (up to the age of 18 or so) looks as if it is suffering from inflammatory change. It is rarely necessary to perform special views of the sacroiliac joints as they show up well on a standard view of the pelvis. This view gives a lot of other information, including the presence of hip disease, pubic symphysitis, and osteitis along the iliac crest and the pubic rami, which can all give important clues to the diagnosis.

(b) *Spine*. As the disease involves the spine, there is a line of advancing inflammation in the paraspinal ligaments. This brings behind it osteoblastic activity which in turn leads to the formation of the typical ligamentous ossification – the syndesmophyte. This is clearly visible on plain X-ray. Contrary to common belief the ossification does not start in the sacrum and work up, but rather starts at the dorsilumbar junction and moves up and down from this site. Therefore spinal X-rays should be centred at D12 if early syndesmophyte formation is being sought. Syndesmophytes are best demonstrated in anterior–posterior views but lateral views will reveal squaring of the vertebral bodies which is the earliest spinal change in AS, as well as identifying erosive changes – the Romanoff lesion. The cervical spine is likely to be involved in progressive cases and should be X-rayed in the lateral projection.

(c) *Other imaging techniques.* There is still debate as to whether bone scans are helpful in diagnosing early sacroilitis. On balance, it does not seem to be a useful technique for this purpose but may be useful in picking up inflammatory change in unusual sites such as the manubrio-sternal joint. By the same token infra-red thermography seems to have little place in the diagnosis of sacroilitis.

Tissue typing

This is placed deliberately at the end of the section on investigation as there is very little, if any, place for using tissue typing in the diagnosis of AS and the related seronegative conditions. The technique is expensive and time-consuming, and there is such a high correlation with radiological sacroilitis that if the X-ray is negative, then the individual is likely not to carry the B-27 antigen. If he or she does, then it is likely that the individual will belong to the 8 per cent or so of the normal population that carries the antigen. It is known that, at the most, only 10 per cent of the B-27 population will have a seronegative arthropathy, and some authors put the figure as low as 1 per cent. This being the case there can be no justification for using tissue typing for anything other than research.

Psoriatic arthritis

Psoriasis is a common skin condition, occurring in about 3 per cent of the population. Something like 15 per cent of these patients will suffer from one of the three forms of specific psoriatic arthritis. As the condition is so common, it is not unusual to see other common forms of arthritis (such as osteoarthritis or seropositive rheumatoid arthritis) as a chance accompaniment of the skin disease. Psoriasis can occur at any age and the psoriatic arthritis may appear at the same time as the skin condition, some time after (which is the most common) or some time later.

Presentation

Mild peripheral disease

This is by far the most common form of psoriatic arthritis. It usually affects the hands and feet, although any joint can be affected. It is differentiated from rheumatoid arthritis by a number of features (including the presence of psoriasis). The first is the involvement of the distal interphalangeal joints in psoriasis. It is important not to confuse distal arthritis with Heberden's nodes in osteoarthritis, which is so common especially in women. The other main difference is the degree of soft tissue swelling that occurs, producing the so-called sausage digit. This form of psoriatic arthritis is benign and non-progressive and usually can be controlled with non-steroidal anti-inflammatory agents. This variety is not associated with the B-27 antigen. It is usual for the arthritis to get worse when the skin lesions deteriorate. The skin disease is normally the mild type with plaques on the elbows, knees and in the scalp, or of geographic distribution. Sometimes the skin lesions are so sparse that they have to be sought with great care in such sites as the umbilicus or natal cleft. When there is distal interphalangeal joint involvement there is likely to be nail pitting or onycholysis – that is thickening of the nail with separation of the nail plate.

Mutilating arthritis

This is an uncommon condition which produces some of the severest joint destruction seen. The psoriasis is usually extensive, often of the *homme rouge* variety. The extensive erosive change may well produce the so-called opera-glass fingers. The amount of bone resorption is such that there is considerable shortening of the phalangeal bones and hence the fingers can be extended and pushed back in like opera-glasses (Figure 2.10). Other joints may be so badly damaged that there is major handicap. Involvement of the cervical spine can be life-threatening. Again this type of arthritis is not associated with the B-27 antigen. This form will require treatment with powerful second-line drugs.

Spondylitis

This group is associated with the B-27 antigen. Apart from the presence of the psoriasis there is little to distinguish the disease from AS, except that the sacroilitis is likely to be asymmetrical. Unlike the other two forms of psoriatic arthritis there seems to be little linkage between the activity of the skin disease and the spondylitis.

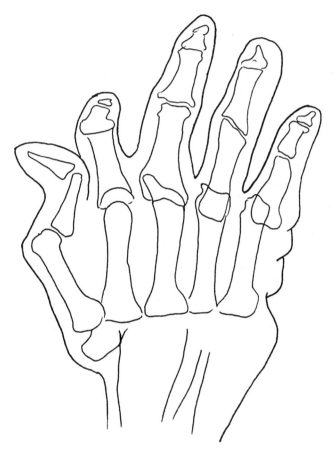

Figure 2.10   X-ray of severe mutilating arthritis in psoriasis

Investigations

Full blood count

(a) *Haemoglobin.* All forms of psoriatic arthritis may show evidence of the anaemia of chronic inflammation.

(b) *Sedimentation rate*. The ESR is likely to be raised in the two types of peripheral disease but like AS itself, in the spondylitic version, the ESR may be normal.

X-rays

X-rays of the hands will show erosive change in the mild disease, not only in the sites seen in rheumatoid arthritis (carpus, ulnar styloid, metacarpophalangeal and proximal interphalangeal joints) but also in the distal interphalangeal joints. In the mutilating disease the classic X-ray appearance is that of the pencil and cup deformity due to extensive remodelling (Figure 2.11). As noted above, in the spondylitic form of the disease, the sacroilitis is likely to be asymmetrical.

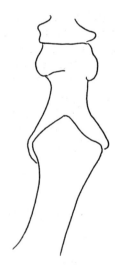

Figure 2.11   Pencil and cup deformity in psoriasis

Reiter's syndrome

This disease is perhaps better called reactive arthritis. The majority of sufferers carry the B-27 antigen and usually it is possible to identify an infective episode and even, on occasion, the causative infective agent. It has been the study of this condition, with its extension to AS itself, which represents one of the most exciting advances in modern medicine.

Presentation

Joints

The arthritis of Reiter's syndrome can be peripheral or spinal. The peripheral disease often affects the lower limbs only, with the metatarsophalangeal, subtalar, ankle and knee joints bearing the brunt of the disease. There is frequently an enthesopathy (which is also seen in AS), which leads to plantar fasciitis leading to pain in the heel, and Achilles tendonitis with pain and swelling behind the ankle. The spinal disease is like mild AS but may be asymmetrical. The joint disease may subside but it is best to be guarded about the prognosis as recurrence is frequent, even if there is not re-exposure to the precipitating factor (see below).

Skin

A variety of mucocutaneous lesions is seen, some of which are quite distinctive. The first is keratodermia blenorrhagica, which is a psoriasis-like rash on the soles of the feet. The other typical lesion is circinate balinitis on the glans penis. This looks like superficial ulceration of the glans and is similar to the aphous ulceration seen in the mouth in Reiter's syndrome.

Occasionally there is a more extensive rash which looks very much like guttate psoriasis and rarely this will become so extensive that it looks like the *homme rouge* stage of psoriasis.

The eye

Conjunctivitis is the commonest eye complication but anterior uveitis can be seen.

The urethra

Urethritis is an almost constant finding. Many patients with Reiter's syndrome have acquired their disease sexually. The Reiter's syndrome is a complication of non-specific urethritis. However, it is now recognised that the majority of patients acquire their disease following dysentery. Even in the post-dysenteric form there is urethritis. This may be noted because of frank discharge or dysuria, but in other forms it will be silent. Urethritis can be tested for by doing a two-glass test. In this, the bladder is emptied first thing in the morning. The first part of the specimen is passed into one glass and the second into the second glass. If urethritis is present the first portion will be obviously cloudier than the second and threads of discharge may be seen in the first glass.

Investigations

Full blood count

(a) *Haemoglobin*. There is likely to be an anaemia or chronic inflammation.

(b) *Sedimentation rate*. The ESR is usually raised in Reiter's syndrome.

Microbiology

(a) *Urethra*. In patients who have acquired their disease sexually there is about a 50 per cent chance of identifying *Chlamydia* in the discharge.

(b) *Bowel*. The syndrome may only come on 1–4 weeks after the dysentery but, where sampling is done at the time of the diarrhoea, a number of organisms may be identified. They include *Salmonella* species, *Shigella* and *Yersinia*.

X-rays

Plain films of the feet may show an exuberant plantar spur, erosion at the site of insertion of the Achilles tendon and erosive change in the small joints of the feet. The pelvic X-ray will show asymmetrical sacroilitis in those patients with spinal disease.

Gut-related arthritis

Both Crohn's disease and ulcerative colitis may be complicated by arthritis.

Presentation

Peripheral arthritis

This problem is one of a large joint arthritis, usually affecting the knees. There tends to be quite large effusions, which are sterile. The arthritis comes and goes with the gut disease and, if the diseased gut is resected, the arthritis usually disappears.

Spondylitis

This looks very much like AS and does not respond to gut resection.

Investigations

There are no special features of the investigation other than the findings on barium enema and the examination of the bowel at sigmoidoscopy or operation. If a patient with peripheral or spinal arthritis complains of abdominal symptoms, it is important to investigate the bowel properly.

Viral Arthritis

Many viruses can precipitate arthralgia or arthritis. Hence arthralgia is commonplace in influenza or the common cold. More importantly, there is the group of reactive arthropathies following viral infection. The best known is rubella but many others have been implicated. Recently the parvovirus (the cause of fifth disease or slapped cheek syndrome) has been shown to be responsible for limited epidemics of arthritis. Most viral arthropathies are limited and will get better after about 6–8 weeks. The diagnosis is often made by watching the course of the disease and by identifying other cases in the community. However, if the diagnosis is considered early enough, blood and stool specimens can be taken as soon as possible and in the convalescent phase, to show a rising titre of antibody to the responsible organism.

CHAPTER 3

PAIN IN THE HAND

Introduction

The hand is the structure which allows man to make use of his considerable intellect. It allows him (and of course her) to manipulate the environment. It is not surprising, therefore, that when there is pain in the hand the doctor is often consulted early. Patients are very concerned about losing hand function, whatever their occupation. Pain may arise from any number of structures but it is arthritis in its many forms that cause the most concern and the most disability.

As with the succeeding chapters, the manifestations of the major diseases in the hand will be described, together with certain localised conditions that are peculiar to the hand. Attention will also be drawn to the special physical signs that are to be found in the hand, which are relevant to more widespread rheumatic disease.

The History

When a patient presents with hand pain a number of questions need to be answered, either in the complaint of the patient or on direct questioning.

1   How long has the pain been present?
2   Is this the first episode or has it occurred before?
3   Where in the hand is the pain?
4   What is the nature of the pain?
5   Is the pain worse at any particular time of day?
6   Is the pain worse on movement?
7   Does the pain limit function?
8   Was there an obvious precipitating cause?
9   Is there stiffness and if so when is it worse?
10   Is there joint swelling?
11   Where is the joint swelling?
12   Are other joints involved?
13   Are there any paraesthesiae?
14   Is there any weakness?
15   Are there any systemic symptoms?
16   Is there a significant past history?
17   Is there a significant family history?
18   What treatment has been tried and has it been effective?

It can be seen that a very thorough history is necessary if mistakes are to be avoided.

The Examination

Once a satisfactory history has been obtained the hand

can be examined. Firstly the hand and wrist should be inspected; then the various joints and the soft tissues are palpated. Next, the patient is asked to demonstrate the range and strength of the various joints and, finally, simple neurological testing is undertaken. For ease of presentation the various parts of the examination are given in tabular form for each part of the hand and wrist. After each table some explanation is added where it is thought helpful.

The nail

Table 3.1   Examination of the nail

Inspection	Palpation	Possible cause
Clubbing	Soft nail beds	Lung, heart and abdominal disease
Koilonychia	Soft nail	Iron deficiency
Splinter haemorrhages	—	Bacterial endocarditis
Pitting	—	Psoriasis
Onycholysis	—	Psoriasis
Pallor	—	Anaemia, liver disease
Absent or much reduced in size	—	Nail-patella syndrome
Nailfold infarcts	Tenderness	Vasculitis
Paronychia	Tenderness	Infection
Bitten	—	Anxiety

Clubbing is an important physical sign. Hypertrophic pulmonary osteoarthropathy can cause pain in the hands and wrists that is indistinguishable from inflammatory arthritis. Clubbing should alert the doctor to the possibility. Pseudoclubbing is frequent and clubbing should only be described as such if there is loss of the nail angle (Figure 3.1) and bogginess of the nail-bed.

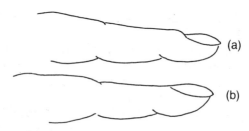

Figure 3.1   (a) Normal nail bed angle, (b) clubbing

Many people have a few pits in their nails but this does not mean that they have psoriasis. The best approach is to count the total number of pits on all the fingernails and if the number exceeds 20, then that is significant.

Dilated nailfold capillaries are typically seen in dermatomyositis but may be present in any of the connective tissues disorders.

The skin

Table 3.2   Examination of the skin

Inspection	Palpation	Cause
Erythema (palmar)	—	Liver disease, rheumatoid arthritis
Erythema	Warm	Inflammation of underlying structure
Pallor	—	Anaemia
Vitiligo	—	Connective tissue disorder
Oedema	Pitting	Joint inflammation
Dusky	—	Raynaud's phenomenon
Subcutaneous tissue loss	Woody feel	Scleroderma
Psoriasis	—	Psoriasis
Vesicles	—	Herpes zoster
Thickened skin	Thickened	(a) Dupuytren's diathesis
		(b) Rheumatoid nodules
		(c) Collodion patches of dermatomyositis
		(d) Occupational callus
Gangrene	—	Vasculitis

Palmar erythema (liver palms) is frequently seen in rheumatoid arthritis.

Vitiligo is a common accompaniment of a wide range of connective tissue disorders and it is always wise to perform an autoantibody screen in patients with the condition.

Pitting oedema is often seen proximally to an inflamed joint, particularly acute gout and acute rheumatoid arthritis.

Raynaud's phenomenon can occur as an idiopathic condition or as a complication of a number of conditions, including rheumatoid arthritis, scleroderma and systemic lupus erythematosus. The condition is discussed further below.

Digital gangrene may be due to vasculitis complicating a connective tissue disease, rheumatoid arthritis or diabetes.

The joints

Table 3.3   Examination of the joints

Inspection	Palpation	Causes
Erythema	Warm, tender	Rheumatoid arthritis
		Other inflammatory arthritides
		Gout
		Pyrophosphate deposition disease
		Acute osteoarthritis
		Septic arthritis
Swelling	Tender	As above plus:
		Nodal osteoarthritis
		Gouty tophi
		Oedema
		Garrod's pads
		Tenosynovitis

Table 3.3 (cont.) Examination of the joints

Inspection	Palpation	Causes
Loss of range	Crepitus	Rheumatoid arthritis Other inflammatory arthritides Osteoarthritis Acute crystal deposition Scleroderma Diabetes Trauma Shoulder–hand syndrome Trigger finger Sepsis
Hypermobility	—	Hypermobility syndrome
Deformity	Crepitus	Rheumatoid arthritis Psoriatic arthritis Advanced gout Trauma Congenital abnormality Nerve lesions
Loss of function	Weakness	Rheumatoid arthritis Other inflammatory arthritides Osteoarthritis Scleroderma Shoulder–hand syndrome Trauma Congenital deformity Neurological lesions

The distribution of the joint disease gives considerable help in making the diagnosis. The main sites in the hand and wrist are given in Table 3.4.

The hand is about function, and it is important to get a feel for how the hand is being used. A simple set of functional tests, such as doing up buttons and writing, are all worth assessing in the clinic. A more formal assessment should be undertaken by the occupational therapist.

Table 3.4 *Distribution of joint disease in the hand*

Site	Disease
Distal interphalangeal	Osteoarthritis
	Psoriasis
	Gout
Proximal interphalangeal	Rheumatoid arthritis
	Osteoarthritis
Metacarpo-phalangeal	Rheumatoid arthritis
	Haemochromatosis
First carpometacarpal	Osteoarthritis
Carpus	Rheumatoid arthritis
	Seronegative arthritis
	Sepsis
Wrist	Rheumatoid arthritis
	Gout
	Pyrophosphate deposition disease
	Trauma
	Hypertrophic pulmonary osteoarthropathy

The muscles

Table 3.5 *Examination of the muscles*

Inspection	Palpation	Causes
Wasting	Loss of tone	Carpal tunnel syndrome
		Rheumatoid arthritis
		Lower motor neurone lesions
Weakness	Loss of power	Severe arthritis
		Severe pain from any cause
		Neurological lesions
Fasciculation	—	Motor neurone disease

Small muscle wasting is a common physical sign in inflammatory arthritis. If a muscle is not used it rapidly wastes and becomes weak. Small muscle wasting in the hand may exaggerate joint swelling.

Although motor neurone disease spares the sensory nerves, spasm in the muscles may be intensely painful.

The nerves

Table 3.6   *Examination of the nerves in the hand*

Lesion	Physical signs	Causes
Carpal tunnel syndrome	Wasting of abductor pollicis brevis (APB) Weakness of APB Blunting to pin-prick, median distribution Positive Tinel's sign Positive Phalen's sign	Rheumatoid arthritis Acromegaly Myxoedema Amyloidosis
Ulnar nerve compression	Wasting of small muscles of the hand Weakness of small muscles of the hand Blunting to pin-prick, ulnar distribution	Arthritis in elbow Arthritis in wrist Elbow trauma
Nerve root compression	Weakness of muscles in the hand (for full list see Table 5.2) Alteration of sensation in root distribution (see Table 5.2) Reduction or loss of appropriate tendon reflexes (Table 5.2)	Cervical spondylosis Rheumatoid arthritis Ankylosing spondylitis Herpes zoster Pathological fracture
Mononeuritis multiplex	Any combination of nerve lesions	Polyarteritis nodosa Diabetes Rheumatoid vasculitis Systemic lupus erythematosus
Peripheral neuropathy	Loss of sensation in glove distribution	Diabetes Rheumatoid vasculitis Systemic lupus erythematosus Vitamin B12 deficiency Multiple sclerosis Toxins Guillain–Barré syndrome Non-metastatic malignant neuropathy Hereditary neuropathies

Carpal tunnel syndrome is a frequent accompaniment of rheumatoid arthritis. Patients will complain of tingling in the hand and probably will not realise that the little finger has been spared until the fact is pointed out to them. The weakness in the abductor pollicis brevis is tested with the hand palm up on a flat surface. The examiner places his index finger on the end of the thumb, with his middle and ring fingers on the belly of the muscle. The patient is then asked to raise the thumb up vertically from the surface and the strength and bulk of the muscle is assessed (Figure 3.2). Patients often try and bring the thumb out sideways when this test is attempted, and they may have to be shown exactly what is required.

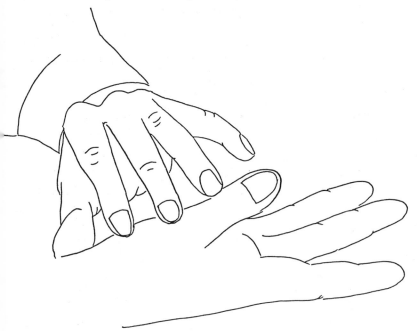

Figure 3.2   Testing the strength of the abductor pollicis brevis

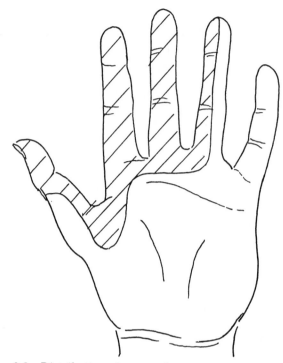

Figure 3.3   Distribution of sensory loss in carpal tunnel syndrome

The blunting of sensation (most usually done with pin-prick) is in the median distribution (Figure 3.3). It must be remembered that variation in the distribution is common and that the whole palm may be supplied by the median nerve or that the ulnar nerve may supply the whole of the ring finger and even the middle finger. In the early stages there may be hypersensitivity rather than loss of sensation in the median distribution. Tinel's sign is performed by lightly percussing the median nerve at the wrist crease. The test is positive if there is the production of paraesthesiae in the median distribution. It is often during the performance of this test that the sparing of the little finger can be demonstrated to the patient. Phalen's test is done by getting the patient to hold the wrist fully flexed for about a minute. This again reproduces the paraesthesiae.

Weakness of the small muscles of the hand in ulnar nerve lesions can be demonstrated in a number of ways. Two simple tests are to get the patient to try to hold onto a card held between the outstretched fingers. The patient is then asked to spread the fingers apart against resistance provided by the examiner (Figure 3.4).

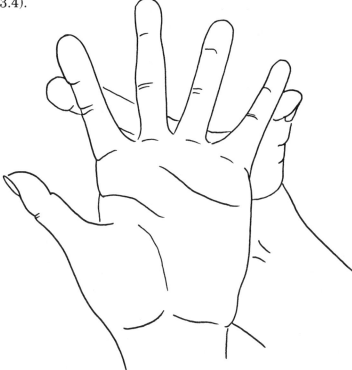

Figure 3.4   Testing intrinsic muscle strength in the hand

If there is a long-standing ulnar nerve lesion the hand develops a classical shape, the 'claw hand'. In this the metacarpophalangeal joints of the ring and little fingers are held in hyperextension, with the interphalangeal joints held in flexion.

A wide range of disorders can produce neurological signs and symptoms in the hand, with pain as an important feature. It is important to look beyond the hand if nerve damage is found or if the patient complains of paraesthesiae.

Investigation of the Hand and Wrist

A number of techniques are available to investigate the hand. In Chapter 2 the investigations appropriate for systemic disease were discussed and will not be repeated here. Rather those investigations that are directly referable to the hand will be considered.

X-rays

The plain film of the hand and wrist is one of the most useful investigations in rheumatology. Table 3.7 lists the common X-ray appearances that may be seen in the painful hand. It is usually sufficient to take just one view, a straight anteroposterior film of both hands on a single plate with the fingers held apart and including the wrist. Special views of the scaphoid may be necessary if a fracture is suspected but other views, such as the cricket ball, rarely give any extra information.

Table 3.7   X-ray appearances in the hand and wrist

Lesion	Site	Causes
Osteoporosis	Generalised	Disuse Sepsis Steroids
	Patchy	Sudek's atrophy Shoulder–hand syndrome

Erosions	Peri-articular
	Distal interphalangeal
	  joints
		Inflammatory arthritis
		Psoriasis
		Gout
		(Osteoarthritis – the
		  cysts may mimic
		  erosions)

	Proximal
	  interphalangeal
	  joints
		Rheumatoid arthritis
		Psoriasis

	Metacarpophalangeal joints	Rheumatoid arthritis Psoriasis Haemochromatosis
	First carpometacarpal joints	Osteoarthritis
	Carpus	Rheumatoid arthritis Seronegative arthritis Sepsis Juvenile chronic arthritis
	Ulnar styloid	Rheumatoid arthritis Seronegative arthritis
Loss of joint space	Distal interphalangeal joints	Psoriasis Osteoarthritis Gout

	Proximal
	  interphalangeal
	  joints
		Rheumatoid arthritis
		Osteoarthritis
		Psoriasis
		Sepsis

	Metacarpophalangeal joints	Rheumatoid arthritis Seronegative arthritis Haemochromatosis Sepsis
	First carpometacarpal joint	Osteoarthritis
	Carpus	Rheumatoid arthritis Seronegative arthritis Sepsis Juvenile chronic arthritis

Table 3.7 (cont.) X-ray appearances in the hand and wrist

Lesion	Site	Causes
Deformity	Distal interphalangeal joints	Osteoarthritis Psoriasis Trauma
	Proximal interphalangeal joints	Rheumatoid arthritis Osteoarthritis
	Metacarpophalangeal joints	Rheumatoid arthritis (ulnar drift) Psoriasis (pen and cup) Haemochromatosis
	Carpus and wrist	Rheumatoid arthritis Psoriasis Juvenile chronic arthritis Trauma (Colles' fracture)
Cysts	Distal interphalangeal joints	Osteoarthritis Gout
	Proximal interphalangeal joints	Osteoarthritis Rheumatoid arthritis (pre-erosive)
	Metacarpophalangeal joints	Rheumatoid arthritis (pre-erosive)
	Carpus and wrist	Rheumatoid arthritis (pre-erosive, geodes) Osteoarthritis Pyrophosphate deposition
Loss of bone	Distal phalangeal bone	Trauma Scleroderma
	Other sites	Trauma Tumours Sepsis
Increased density	Scaphoid	Aseptic necrosis (following ununited fracture)
	Other sites	Paget's disease of bone Tumour
Increased distal tufts	—	Acromegaly
Periosteal reaction	Any	Hypertrophic pulmonary osteoarthropathy Sepsis

Table 3.7 (cont.)   X-ray appearances in the hand and wrist

Lesion	Site	Causes
Periosteal reaction		Bleeding disorders
		Juvenile chronic arthritis
		Hyperparathyroidism (resorption)
		Thyroid acropathy
Soft tissue calcification	Fingers	Scleroderma
		Dermatomyositis (children)
	Joints	Pyrophosphate deposition
		Gout
		Haemochromatosis
	Blood vessels	Diabetes
		Atherosclerosis

To describe an erosion it is important to demonstrate an actual breach in the cortex of the bone. Although the ulnar styloid does not articulate with any other bone in the human hand there is a synovial remnant present and this is frequently inflamed early in rheumatoid arthritis; hence the first erosion may well occur at this site. If erosive change is being used to follow the course of rheumatoid arthritis, progression should only be described if new erosions are appearing. Old erosions tend to get bigger just from 'wear and tear'.

The typical lesion of osteoarthritis is a bone cyst but the walls may collapse to produce an appearance very similar to an erosion.

Infection, either acute or chronic, typically crosses the joint, giving osteoporosis, loss of joint space and periosteal reaction.

In rheumatoid arthritis the pannus may invade the bone to create a cyst. Sometimes these reach large proportions and are then called geodes after cystic rock formations containing a lining of crystals seen in geology. These geodes may suddenly collapse, producing a rapid increase in pain and deformity.

Electrodiagnosis

The electromyograph (EMG) is of particular importance in the diagnosis of neurological lesions involving the hand. Typically EMGs can be used to measure the latency of the median nerve at the wrist and elbow. The latency is the time taken for an electrical impulse to travel from the point at which the nerve is stimulated to the muscle being studied (the abductor pollicis brevis, in the case of the median nerve) and for a contraction to occur which can be picked up by the surface electrode. The upper limit of normal for the median nerve is 4.5 milliseconds. If it is longer than this then carpal tunnel compression is proven unless the conduction velocity in the whole nerve is grossly slowed. This can be shown by stimulating the nerve at the elbow, subtracting the two latencies to measure the time taken for the impulse to travel along the segment of nerve. This distance is measured and the conduction velocity calculated. The normal value is in excess of 45 metres/second. Sensory latencies and conduction velocities can also be found by using stimulators that slip over a finger, the recording electrode being placed at the wrist and the elbow. The size (amplitude) of the impulse can also be measured, and this gives the earliest evidence of nerve damage.

The use of needle electrodes allows evidence of denervation to be sought, as well as looking for the spontaneous discharges of motor neurone disease, etc. Denervation can also be assessed by doing strength/

duration curves using a simple muscle stimulator alone.

Thermography

Until recently this has been mainly a research tool but many hospitals now have the equipment. It has two main uses in the hand. The first is to identify hot joints. Thermography measures heat emission from the body and a quantitative index of joint inflammation can be obtained. This index can be used to follow the course of disease and the influence of treatment.

The second use is to define vasospasm in Raynaud's phenomenon. Normally when the hand is placed in cold water and then removed the hand cools in the water, but when it is removed it does not just heat up. Instead there is a fairly marked hyperaemia, with a temperature rise of a couple of degrees centigrade. By way of contrast in Raynaud's phenomenon there is marked vasospasm when the hand is removed from the water, with a considerable drop in temperature of the hand. It has been found that the vasospasm is severest in scleroderma. The water does not need to be very cold to perform this test, 20 degrees centigrade being quite cool enough.

Bone scan

Bone scan, using technetium, can be used to detect the presence of synovitis at a very early stage, before there are any definite changes on X-ray. Scans are also a useful way of detecting the changes associated with metabolic bone disease.

Specific Conditions in the Hand and Wrist

The way that specific conditions affect the hand and wrist will now be discussed. With the systemic conditions, such as rheumatoid arthritis, the treatment will be discussed in Chapter 12. In more localised conditions the treatment will be discussed here. This pattern will be repeated in succeeding chapters.

Rheumatoid arthritis (RA)

RA affects the hand frequently and early. It is also a common condition and hence it is important to know how it can affect the hand. Although the feet are often affected first, it is usually hand disease that brings the patient to the doctor because of the functional implications of arthritic hands. In the acute stage the hand may well be swollen, with pitting oedema. Pain is an almost constant feature and there will be morning stiffness which, in the acute stage, can last all day. There is likely to be swelling of the proximal interphalangeal and metacarpophalangeal joints, as well as the wrist. Although symmetrical, often the dominant hand is affected more. Sometimes just one or two joints are affected, the more widespread disease not appearing for many months or even years. As time goes by the boggy joint swelling will give way to joint disruption and deformity if the disease is not controlled.

There are several typical deformities in the hand. The most common is ulnar drift. The normal action of the finger flexors is to pull the hand into ulnar drift on gripping. In RA this tendency is made worse by the

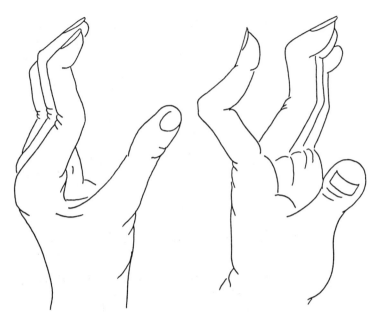

Figure 3.5a   Swan-neck   *Figure 3.5b   Boutonnière*

flexor tendons slipping medially, producing a bowstring effect. As this is a dynamic deformity splinting
will not help. Careful examination of a hand with ulnar
drift will usually reveal that there is a radial deformity
of the wrist. The fingers show two main types of
deformity. The first is swan-necking, in which there is
hyperextension of the proximal interphalangeal joint
and flexion of the distal interphalangeal joint (Figure
3.5a). The boutonnière deformity is fixed flexion of the
proximal interphalangeal joint with hyperextension of
the distal interphalangeal joint (Figure 3.5b). The
thumb develops a characteristic problem, the Z-
deformity. It actually allows better function in the
hand by bringing the side of the thumb into opposition
with the side of the hand, allowing a modified pinch
grip (Figure 3.6).

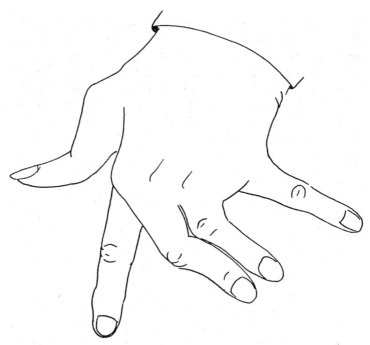

*Figure 3.6   Z-deformity of the thumb
(with ulnar drift of the fingers).*

The wrist will be considerably disrupted in late disease with virtual resorption of the carpus and an unstable flexion deformity. Such a wrist puts the finger flexors at a considerable mechanical disadvantage. It is therefore always worth considering putting the wrist in a simple elasticated splint and even seeking surgical fusion.

Small muscle wasting is common, secondary to the joint disease, and this may aggravate poor hand function. If the inflammatory process involves the extensor tendons there is the risk of rupture. This leads to 'dropped' fingers, the little finger usually being the first to go, followed by the ring, middle and even index fingers. Functionally this is not necessarily a serious problem, although the dropped finger or fingers may get in the way. If the hand is splinted with the fingers in extension healing can take place spontaneously but surgery is usually needed to repair the tendon or tendons. This should be done quickly as there is a tendency for the tendons to retract. The other problem with tendons is the formation of nodules, especially in the flexor tendons in the palm, producing a trigger finger. In this complication the finger flexes without difficulty but when extension is attempted the finger becomes stuck and has to be forced back, often with a palpable snap, which can be painful. These usually respond to local steroid injections. A ganglion is a cystic outgrowth from a tendon and these are seen quite frequently in RA around the wrist.

As stated above, carpal tunnel syndrome is a frequent accompaniment of RA and any worsening of pain or loss of function should raise the possibility of nerve compression. Weakness can also occur because of spinal cord compression due to an unstable neck (see Chapter 5) or more rarely due to mononeuritis multiplex. This last-named complication is a consequence of vasculitis. This may show up in the form of nailfold lesions or bigger areas of infarction. Raynaud's phenomenon may be obvious.

Recently it has been suggested that seronegative RA may have a different pattern of joint involvement, with predominently carpal erosive change.

Psoriatic arthritis (PSA)

As explained in Chapter 2 there are two main forms of

peripheral PSA. The mild disease is a symmetrical polyarthritis which affects all the small joints in the hand. The dorsal interphalangeal joints may be particularly affected and under these circumstances there is often pitting of the nails. The course is benign and there are not likely to be any signs apart from some mild swelling of the joints.

The mutilating form of the disease produces the most bizarre deformities of the hand. Opera-glass fingers were described earlier, and these are accompanied by the pen and cup appearances on X-ray. As with the other seronegative arthritides there is a distinct tendency for the wrist and carpus to bear the brunt of the disease. The grossly unstable wrist that is produced seriously interferes with the function of the hand flexors. With this variety of PSA the skin disease is frequently aggressive and the hands can be completely covered with severe psoriasis, with considerable nail involvement.

Osteoarthritis (OA)

Generalised nodal OA is characterised in the hand by three cardinal features. These are (a) Heberden's nodes, (b) Bouchard's nodes, and (c) the square hand.

Heberden's nodes occur on the distal interphalangeal joint. They are painful as they grow but once they are mature they become pain-free. They can become very inflamed in early stages and the patient will complain of throbbing pain. At this stage they may even discharge glairy fluid. The nodes are, in fact, bony cysts whose walls can collapse, giving rise to deformity of the finger-ends. As Heberden's nodes are self-limiting they usually do not cause too much long-term trouble but can be disabling for a typist or professional musician.

Bouchard's node is a bone cyst occurring in the proximal interphalangeal joint rather than the distal. Again they are self-limiting. Patients with prominent Bouchard's nodes are often mistaken for RA sufferers, especially as morning stiffness, albeit for a few minutes only, may also be prominent. However, the presence of Heberden's nodes and a square hand, together with negative blood tests and the typical cystic X-rays, should make the diagnosis easy. If Bouchard's or Heberden's nodes are very painful they can be injected with small doses of corticosteroids, avoiding triamcinalone as in such superficial sites obvious skin atrophy is likely.

The square hand appearance is due to degeneration in the first carpometacarpal joint. The joint is tender and tasks involving a power grip are likely to be painful and even make the patient drop things. Unlike Heberden's and Bouchard's nodes this abnormality is not particularly self-limiting. Steroid injection can help, as will a small polythene splint to stabilise the joint, but a number of these patients come to surgery to have the trapezium either removed or replaced with a silastic prosthesis.

Gout

Acute attacks of gout are common in the wrist, while tophi may well form in the finger-ends. As with gout elsewhere the acute attack comes on suddenly, often overnight. The joint becomes exquisitely painful. The patient will not tolerate the joint being touched. The overlying skin is red, hot and dry.

Tophi will form around the distal interphalangeal joint and may resemble Heberden's nodes but the white monosodium urate crystals are usually obvious. It is not unusual for a tophus to discharge its contents chronically in long-standing patients with high levels of serum urate. The treatment of gout is discussed in Chapter 12.

Calcium pyrophosphate deposition disease (CPPD)

CPPD often attacks the hands. In this site attacks of pseudo-gout are unusual, the major manifestation being accelerated OA. There is an association with Heberden's nodes and the clinical picture may be indistinguishable from OA. However the finding of calcification in the triangular ligament of the wrist will show that CPPD is the underlying cause and that the prognosis is not quite so good as with OA. Treatment at the moment is entirely symptomatic, including steroid injection.

Haemochromatosis

This is a rare condition in which there is abnormal iron metabolism. The iron is laid down in the liver, leading to cirrhosis; the pancreas, leading to diabetes mellitus; the heart, leading to cardiomyopathy; and the skin, leading to the typical bronze pigmentation. It is usually seen in middle-aged men. In the joints calcium pyrophosphate is laid down and marked degenerative changes occur in the index and middle finger metacarpal joints, giving a very characteristic appearance.

Raynaud's disease

When Raynaud's phenomenon occurs without an underlying cause it can correctly be called idiopathic Raynaud's disease. This is probably the commonest cause of symptomatic Raynaud's phenomenon. The patient will complain of pain in the hands in cold weather, together with some swelling of the fingers. The patient will also report that the hands change colour, ranging from red through white to blue. A similar set of symptoms may occur in very hot conditions. Treatment is unsatisfactory. Patients should be advised to avoid extremes of temperature and to wear warm socks and gloves. Vasodilators are not particularly helpful and sympathectomy, either chemical or surgical, is generally fairly short-lived in its effect. Recent studies with nifedipine have been encouraging in selected patients.

Systemic lupus erythematosus (SLE)

SLE frequently affects the hand. Among the manifestations that may be seen is a relatively painful but non-deforming arthritis, swan-necking of the fingers, especially in coloured patients, peripheral neuropathy, and non-specific rash. SLE is discussed fully in Chapter 2.

Scleroderma

As mentioned in Chapter 2, scleroderma is a spectrum of diseases, ranging from the benign CRST syndrome to the more sinister progressive systemic sclerosis. The hand demonstrates many of the physical signs. The patient may well complain of Raynaud's phenomenon and also a mild sinovitis. Examination of the hand will show a number of physical signs. There will be dilatation of capillaries in the nailbed. There will be loss of the pulps of the fingers and a woody feeling to the skin. There will be loss of sweating and telangiectasia may be seen. In advanced cases there will be loss of extension of the fingers and with acrolysis there will be loss of the end of one or more fingers.

Dermatomyositis

This condition shows itself by dilatation of nailbed capillaries, collodion patches on the knuckles, a variety of non-specific rashes and a mild synovitis. As the weakness is mainly proximal it is most unusual for the hand to be weak.

Hypertrophic pulmonary osteoarthropathy (HPOA)

HPOA is most commonly seen with carcinoma of the lung. The periosteal reaction affects the ends of the radius and ulna and the metacarpal and phalangeal bones. Not infrequently this mimics an inflammatory arthritis. However, the presence of clubbing will lead to the diagnosis. For reasons that are not entirely clear the condition can be cured by vagotomy, even if the underlying cause is untreatable, as it frequently is with carcinoma of the lung.

Sepsis

Because the hand is exposed to so many environmental hazards it is a frequent site of infection. This includes acute bacterial infection from penetration injuries, metastatic infection from skin lesions, such as paronychia, and tuberculous dactylitis. When the joints are involved there is likely to be considerable joint and bone destruction; hence it is important not to overlook the possibility of infection.

It is also important to remember the possibility of a foreign body. A special case is that of the intra-articular plant thorn which can lead to a chronic synovitis which will not resolve until the plant material is removed.

Diabetes will predispose to infection. This must always be borne in mind when a diabetic develops a painful joint.

Algodystrophy

There are a number of regionally painful conditions that are known by a variety of names, including Sudeck's atrophy, reflex sympathetic dystrophy syndrome, shoulder–hand syndrome, causalgia and algodystrophy. All these conditions are marked by unremitting pain. Causalgia is pain without any other physical signs, but the others have a variety of signs and may be regarded as synonymous. In the hand there will be discoloration of the skin, which is often blotchy. There is likely to be some swelling. The skin is hypersensitive and the patient will usually protect the hand from any contact. An X-ray will show patchy osteoporosis. In the shoulder–hand syndrome the condition complicates a painful, stiff shoulder from whatever cause. Sudeck's atrophy seems to come on after minor injury to the hand (or foot).

Treatment needs to be vigorous. In the shoulder–hand syndrome it is important to treat the painful shoulder (see Chapter 4). Sympathetic blockade is potentially curative and this can be achieved in a number of ways, including intravenous guanethidine block. Patients with these conditions are probably best managed in a specialist pain clinic.

Trauma

Trauma is most properly dealt with in an orthopaedic text. One traumatic lesion worth mentioning is the fracture of the scaphoid. This is a notoriously difficult fracture to identify and may not show on X-ray initially. If pain remains in the wrist and there is tenderness in the anatomical snuffbox the scaphoid should be X-rayed again. The second film may well show the fracture. Non-union is frequent because of the poor blood supply of the distal portion of the bone. Non-union will inevitably lead to aseptic necrosis and severe osteoarthritis, with considerable disability.

Ganglia

These are common around the wrist and cause little trouble apart from being unsightly. However, there is one circumstance when they are very troublesome, and that is when they form in the flexor tendon of the thumb. Here they form hard, tender nodules which can be very painful. On examination a hard tender lump, like a lead shot, will be felt over the palmar surface of the saddle joint. If the pain is persistent, it is best removed surgically.

Tenosynovitis

Tendon sheaths can become inflammed, producing pain when the muscle is used. Typically there is tenderness over the tendon and on movement there will be crepitus. Practically any tendon can be involved. One special circumstance is Quervain's stenosing tenovaginitis. This involves the tendons of extensor pollicis brevis and abductor pollicis longus. There is pain on moving the thumb out sideways from the palm.

Tenosynovitis is probably best treated by local steroid injections. It is wisest to avoid using triamcinolone, and care must be taken not to place the steroid into the tendon itself, as rupture is likely.

CHAPTER 4

PAIN IN THE SHOULDER AND ELBOW

Introduction

The shoulder is an important mobility joint which allows the hand to be placed in a wide variety of places. Hence it allows a person to put food to the mouth, wipe the perineum, and reach up to shelves; it also assists with throwing. Clearly any condition that affects shoulder mobility is potentially serious. There are a number of specific conditions that affect the shoulder.

The elbow acts as simple hinge, although supination and pronation partly take place at the elbow. There are few specific problems associated with the elbow, except epicondylitis. The bulk of this chapter deals with the shoulder, therefore, but epicondylitis will be mentioned at the end.

The History

Certain features need to be brought out in the history

when a patient presents with shoulder pain.

1 How long has the pain been present?
2 Is this the first episode or has it occurred before?
3 Are both shoulders involved?
4 Is the pain there only on movement, or does it occur at rest?
5 Does the pain disturb sleep?
6 Is there limitation of range?
7 Was there an obvious precipitating cause?
8 Is there stiffness and, if so, when is it worse?
9 Is there any swelling of the joint?
10 Are other joints (including the neck) involved?
11 Are there any paraesthesiae?
12 Is there any weakness?
13 Are there any systemic symptoms?
14 How old is the patient?
15 Is there a significant past history?
16 Is there a significant family history?
17 What treatment has been tried and has it been effective?

Perhaps it is worth adding to this list an enquiry about what the patient means by the shoulder. Shoulder pain is a term used, by the patient, not only for the shoulder joint itself but for the whole of the upper part of the back. Conversely pain in the upper arm (around the deltoid insertion) is often not recognised as shoulder pain.

The Examination

After the history has been obtained the shoulder can be

examined. It is important to examine the shoulder with the patient properly undressed and, if possible, standing. Total elevation of the shoulder is impossible if dressed and sitting. The general shape and symmetry of the shoulders should be noted, as well as any swellings or muscle wasting. The range of each shoulder is then examined. Wherever possible the ranges should be accurately measured and the results charted. The elements of the examination are given in Table 4.1.

Table 4.1   Examination of the shoulder

Physical sign	Site	Cause
Swelling	Anterior shoulder	Rheumatoid arthritis
		Pyrophosphate deposition
		Sepsis
	Upper arm	Ruptured long head of biceps
Wasting	Generalised	Rheumatoid arthritis
		Osteoarthritis
		Neurological disease
	Deltoid	Neuralgic amyotrophy
Tenderness	Anterior shoulder	Rheumatoid arthritis
		Osteoarthritis
		Bicipital tendonitis
	Posterior shoulder	Fibromyalgia
	Deltoid insertion	Referred shoulder pain
Pain on movement	All movements (not all need be involved)	Rheumatoid arthritis
		Seronegative arthritis
		Osteoarthritis
		Capsulitis
		Fracture
		Malignancy
		Bleeding disorders
	Abduction	Painful arc syndrome
Loss of range	All movements (not all need be involved)	Rheumatoid arthritis
		Osteoarthritis
		Seronegative arthritis
		Frozen shoulder
		Malignancy
		Fracture
		Bleeding disorders

Unless there is significant muscle wasting it is unusual to notice much swelling in the shoulder. The joint is very loose (to allow the wide range of movement) and visible swelling requires a considerable effusion to be present.

Tenderness across the back of the shoulders, with or without palpable nodules, is the classical physical sign in fibromyalgia. This condition is discussed fully in Chapter 5.

Tenderness at or near the deltoid insertion, together with pain on movement at this site, is due to referred pain from the shoulder itself, the skin innervation being the same as the shoulder, the circumflex. There is little point in giving local treatment to the site, the pain going when the shoulder is treated.

Pain on movement is one of the most important physical signs in the shoulder. In mild arthritis or periarthritis it is usual for only one or two movements to be painful, e.g. internal rotation in capsulitis. Women tend to notice this first because of the difficulty of putting on the bra. The painful arc is a classical sign in the shoulder. The shoulder is pain-free at rest but as it is abducted pain starts at about 45 degrees and is felt until the shoulder gets to 120 degrees (Figure 4.1). In total elevation the shoulder is again pain-free but the pain is felt in the same range on lowering the arm.

Limitation of range is again important to define. As assessment of progress of treatment depends on having a proper measure of the range, which is recorded, it is important to get into the habit of doing this. Internal rotation is best measured by noting how high up the back the tip of the thumb can be placed, recorded as the vertebra reached. Goniometers are difficult to use with the shoulder; hence it is usual to estimate the values, but with experience this can be accurate.

It is important to examine the neck carefully in

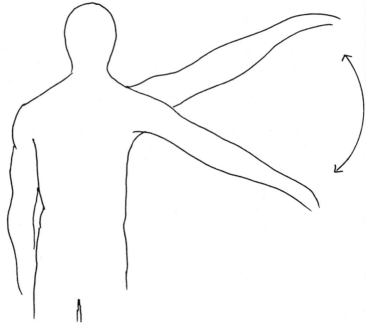

Figure 4.1   Painful arc syndrome

patients complaining of shoulder pain, to exclude a more widespread polyarthritis and examine the breasts in women (because of the possibility of secondary deposits from a carcinoma).

Investigation of Pain in the Shoulder

The detailed investigation of the systemic conditions is given in Chapter 2. The items mentioned here refer specifically to the shoulder.

Blood tests

(a) *Sedimentation rate.* The ESR (and the equivalent non-specific tests) can be used as a screening test in patients with apparently uncomplicated capsulitis. It is especially useful in patients over the age of 55 complaining of shoulder pain and a lot of morning stiffness, the diagnosis of polymyalgia rheumatica coming to mind. However, it will also alert the doctor to the possibility of inflammatory polyarthritis and malignant disease.

(b) *Alkaline phosphatase.* Bone destruction, including myeloma, can cause a rise in the alkaline phosphatase, as can Paget's disease of bone which occasionally occurs around the shoulder. The addition of acid phosphatase will exclude prostatic secondaries in men.

(c) *Immunological tests.* The rheumatoid factor and an auto-antibody screen should be considered if there is any likelihood of systemic arthritis.

X-rays

(a) *Plain films.* These are often disappointing in shoulder pain. They may reveal evidence of osteophytes, erosions and loss of joint space in the various types of arthritis but often they are normal. Calcification in the supraspinatus tendon or subacromial bursa may be seen in painful arc syndrome. In the painful shoulder associated with stroke, subluxation of the head of the humerus may be observed. Bone disease, especially malignant deposits and pathological fracture, may often be shown up. However, in the simple painful conditions X-rays are of little use and should only be done if the disease does not follow its expected course. An ESR is a more useful (and cheaper) test.

(b) *Bone scan*. If bone disease, particularly secondary carcinoma, is suspected this is a 'best buy' investigation, showing up lesions long before they are visible on the plain film.

Aspiration of joint fluid

When there is an obvious effusion this should be aspirated both for diagnostic and therapeutic purposes. Shoulder fluid is often thicker than that seen in the knee, and may be more difficult to aspirate. All samples obtained should be sent for culture and should also be examined for crystals. It should be noted that gout is virtually never seen in the shoulder and hence only pyrophosphate crystals will normally be found.

Electrodiagnosis

The deltoid is a frequent muscle sampled in suspected muscle disease (such as dermatomyositis). This muscle can also become involved in an uncommon complication of the painful shoulder, neuralgic amyotrophy which appears to be a reflex denervation in response to the severe pain. This will show up as partial denervation on both EMG and strength-duration studies.

Specific conditions in the shoulder

Rheumatoid arthritis (RA)

The shoulder is frequently involved in RA. It can be particularly disabling as the joint tends to become limited quickly, thus preventing simple tasks such as doing up the bra, combing the hair or wiping the bottom. As with all painful shoulder conditions, night pain is a feature and this adds significantly to loss of sleep and hence general malaise.

It should be remembered that shoulder movement does not just occur at the glenohumeral joint, and that a lot of the abduction in particular comes from the scapula. Thus even with an almost completely fused shoulder joint quite a lot of movement is still possible.

Seronegative arthritis

Shoulder involvement is common in ankylosing spondylitis (AS) adding to the general loss of mobility of the trunk and neck in advanced cases. Inflammation of the acromio- and sternoclavicular joints are common in AS and this will further embarrass the shoulder joint.

The mutilating variety of psoriatic arthritis can produce very severe shoulder destruction.

Connective tissue diseases

Shoulder involvement is not a feature of this group

particularly, with the exception of dermatomyositis and polymyositis which can present as marked shoulder weakness.

Polymyalgia rheumatica (PMR)

This is a condition of late middle age (over 55 years in 98 per cent of patients) characterised by pain in the shoulder girdle (and to a lesser extent the pelvic girdle); marked morning stiffness, general malaise and a raised ESR. It is usually described as a syndrome as it can herald a number of systemic conditions. About 10 per cent go on to develop rheumatoid arthritis (which is the most important differential diagnosis) and another 5 per cent develop malignant disease, especially multiple myeloma. Something like 20 per cent have the condition as a complication of, or a prodrome to, temporal arteritis. For this reason alone it is an important diagnosis to make.

A mild synovitis is common, especially in the shoulders, and this may persist after the main symptoms have been suppressed by steroids, requiring steroid injection (see below).

Temporal artery biopsy is not a particularly helpful investigation as false positives and negatives are common.

Temporal arteritis should be suspected if there is a history of visual disturbance, temporal headaches or facial pain on talking or eating. Unless treatment is undertaken swiftly blindness or stroke may intervene.

Treatment is with prednisolone. It is usual to start with 10 mg daily in uncomplicated PMR but if temporal arteritis is suspected, then 20 or 30 mg is probably safer. The response is usually dramatic, the symptoms going within 48 hours, many patients saying they are better with the first tablet. Once the symptoms have disappeared and the ESR returned to normal levels the steroids can be slowly reduced to the minimum dose that keeps the patient under control. Some cases will go into remission in 2–4 years, but this is not as common as most texts suggest and even when remission has occurred relapse is common.

Osteoarthritis (OA)

Previous injury or inflammatory disease in the shoulder can lead to OA. As the joint is non-weight-bearing the condition is not that common. There is a variety of very destructive OA, called Milwaukee shoulder, that has been linked to apatite deposition. Aseptic necrosis is also seen and the shoulder is one of the sites of caisson disease seen in divers.

Calcium pyrophosphate deposition disease (CPPD)

The shoulder is a common site for CPPD. Gout, on the other hand, is almost unknown. CPPD can cause a most destructive arthritis in the shoulder, and when it does the typical calcification in the cartilage will disappear. It will be apparent in the knee and other sites. Treatment is symptomatic.

Capsulitis

This is a term used to describe inflammation in the

periarticular structures, leading to pain in the joint. Although voluntary movement may be limited by pain, passive movement is full. The onset can be sudden but often there is no obvious precipitating factor. Bilateral capsulitis is common but when it occurs it is sensible to exclude neck disease. Night pain is a common problem and can be debilitating. If the shoulder is not kept moving a frozen shoulder can result.

Treatment consists of analgesia and injection. A simple analgesic or a non-steroidal anti-inflammatory agent should be used, particularly at night. At this stage, the patient should be encouraged to keep the shoulder moving, within the limits of pain, to prevent a frozen shoulder. A long-acting steroid injection given intra-articularly will usually resolve the pain, although it may need to be repeated (Figure 4.2)

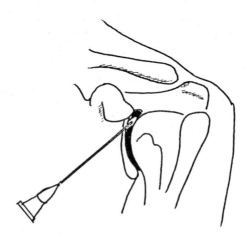

Figure 4.2 Injecting the shoulder by the anterior route

Frozen shoulder

This is sometimes called adhesive capsulitis and can be regarded as a more severe form of capsulitis. The joint range is limited both passively and actively. It is inevitably painful, with night pain a particular problem.

Treatment is again analgesics and steroid injection, but to this should be added physiotherapy to help increase the range of movement. Most cases resolve if properly treated.

Bicipital tendonitis

The bicipital tendon runs through the capsule of the shoulder and can become inflamed and painful. The tendon will be painful and there will be pain on resisted supination of the forearm, with the elbow flexed.

Treatment is with steroid injection, but care must be taken not to inject the tendon itself as rupture can occur. This can also occur spontaneously. Although the lump in the upper arm is quite alarming for the patient, it is not functionally important.

Painful arc syndrome

As described above the painful arc syndrome is caused by the deposition of hydroxyapatite in the subacromial bursa or supraspinatus tendon. The condition is treated by subacromial steroid injection (Figure 4.3).

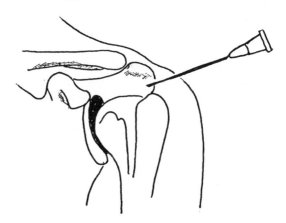

Figure 4.3   Injecting the sub-acromial bursa

Fibromyalgia

This condition is described in full in Chapter 5. It may present as pain in the shoulder, with trigger spots and palpable 'nodules' above the shoulder blades. Although this condition usually complicates cervical spine irritation, it may follow capsulitis.

Stroke

In patients with a dense stroke painful shoulder is common. It may be made worse if the patient is having speech problems, as he may be unable to explain that it is shoulder pain that is causing distress. Examination will show subluxation of the head of the humerus which can be confirmed on X-ray. The joint can be injected to relieve pain, a sling given to hold the humerus in place and the physiotherapist should work to improve tone around the joint.

The Elbow

The number of specific problems associated with the elbow is fairly limited. Rheumatoid arthritis can disrupt the joint and osteoarthritis may occur after injury. Because the ulnar nerve runs in the olecranon groove it is subject to injury and can lead to symptoms of ulnar neuritis in the hand.

Epicondylitis

The only important condition of the elbow is epicondylis. If the lateral epicondyle is involved it is called tennis elbow and if the medial, golfer's elbow.

In tennis elbow (the more common of the two) there is pain and tenderness over the lateral epicondyle and putting strain on the extensor muscles, particularly gripping and turning the hand, is painful. In golfer's elbow it is the common flexor origin that is stressed. Pain is felt in the forearm as well as the elbow. The condition may be precipitated by a blow or by repetitive and unusual stress on the muscles concerned.

Treatment is by steroid injection into the area of maximum tenderness, but this is not always successful. Alternative treatments include the use of an epicondylitis splint, thickening the handle of any tool or racket being used, ultrasound, and, in resistant cases, surgical decompression.

CHAPTER 5

PAIN IN THE NECK

Introduction

The neck is the cause of a considerable number of painful conditions. In this chapter the common musculoskeletal problems will be discussed, but it must be remembered that a lot of other structures are found in the neck and that pain felt in this site may arise from the heart (angina), the respiratory tract (laryngitis), the digestive tract (oesophagitis) and from structures such as lymph glands. It is also important to remember that pain arising from the cervical spine may be felt at a distance from the neck itself.

The History

A careful history will allow the doctor to arrive rapidly at a diagnosis of most causes of neck pain. The following questions require answering in a full history.

1   How long has the pain been present?

2   Is this the first episode or has it occurred before?

3   Was the onset sudden or gradual?

4   Where is the pain?

5   Does it radiate anywhere and, if so, where?

6   What is the nature of the pain?

7   Is the pain there all the time?

8   Is the pain worse at any particular time of day?

9   Is the pain worse on moving the head?

10 Does the pain limit function?

11 Is there any loss of range of the neck?

12 Are there any paraesthesiae?

13 Is there weakness anywhere?

14 Was there a precipitating cause?

15 Are any other joints (including the lumbar spine) involved?

16 Are there any symptoms of systemic disease?

17 Is there a significant past history?

18 Is there a significant family history?

19 What treatment has been tried and has it been effective?

The Examination

Once a full history has been taken the patient can be examined. The symmetry of the head position should be noted and then the range checked. Tender areas in the neck and upper back should be sought, as well as any palpable 'nodules'. The strength of the muscles in the neck and arms is tested, as well as the sensation and tendon reflexes. It is wise to check that the plantar responses are down-going. As a rule a general examination should be carried out, especially if the pain or the clinical course have any unusual features. The main features of the examination of the neck are given in Table 5.1.

Table 5.1 Examination of the neck

Physical sign	Site	Cause
Asymmetry	Head	Torticollis Ankylosing spondylitis Psoriasis Muscle weakness Collapsed vertebra(e)
Loss of range	Any movement of the neck (not all need be involved)	Ankylosing spondylitis Other seronegative arthritides Rheumatoid arthritis Juvenile chronic arthritis Cervical spondylosis Disc lesion Ligamentous lesions Torticollis Trauma (including whiplash) Malignant disease
Tenderness	Posterior neck Across the back	Inflammatory arthritis Cervical spondylosis Malignant disease Fibromyalgia
Pain on movement	Any movement of the neck (not all need be involved)	Rheumatoid arthritis Ankylosing spondylitis Other seronegative arthritides Juvenile chronic arthritis Cervical spondylosis Disc lesions Ligamentous lesions Acute torticollis Malignant disease Trauma
Weakness	Neck	Dermatomyositis hand polymyositis Myasthenia gravis Other neurological disease

Table 5.1 (cont.)   Examination of the neck

Physical sign	Site	Cause
	Both arms	Cord lesion, i.e.
		Trauma
		Central disc protrusion
		Cervical spondylosis
		Rheumatoid arthritis
		Malignant collapse
	One arm	Nerve root compression, i.e.
		Rheumatoid arthritis
		Cervical disc
		Spondylosis
		Other neurological disease
Reflex and sensory changes	Arm	Rheumatoid arthritis
		Cervical disc
		Cervical spondylosis

Asymmetry of the neck is most usually due to torticollis, either acute or chronic. In the acute type the sternomastoid on the side of the head towards which the head is being pulled will be contracted but it is pain on attempted rotation in the opposite direction that blocks the movement while in the chronic type the sternomastoid will be hypertrophied, preventing correction of the deformity, with the contralateral muscle atrophied.

Tenderness across the shoulder blades is associated with fibromyalgia (see below). The tenderness is localised and is often accompanied by palpable 'fibrositic nodules'. Another sign which is seen with this syndrome is painful skin pinch roll in the area of the tender spots.

The sensory changes associated with nerve root compression and irritation are shown in Figure 5.1, and the reflex changes in Table 5.2.

Table 5.2   *Cervical root symptoms and signs*

Root	Area of pain	Muscle weakness	Jerk changes
C2	Occiput, over top of head and to forehead	—	—
C3	Neck, jaw and cheek	—	—
C4	Shoulder, supraclavicular and suprascapular areas	—	—
C5	Deltoid area and lateral side of arm	Spinati, deltoid, biceps	Biceps, brachioradialis
C6	Front of arm and lateral portion of hand	Biceps, supinator, wrist extensors	Biceps
C7	Hand, especially index, middle and ring fingers	Triceps, wrist flexors	Triceps
C8	Medial portion of hand and forearm	Finger and thumb flexors, thumb extensors and abductors	—
T1	Medial side of arm	Intrinsic hand muscles	—
T2	Medial side of upper arm and axilla, upper pectoral and mid-scapula areas	—	—

Investigation of the Painful Neck

Blood tests

(a) *Sedimentation rate.* The ESR is a useful screening test to exclude serious or systemic disease.

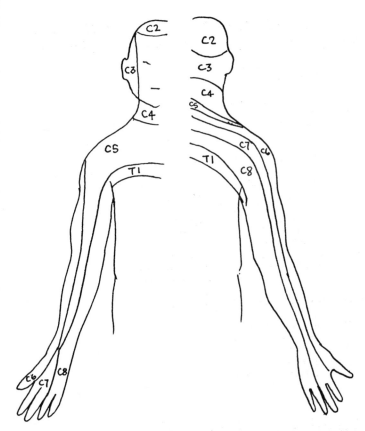

Figure 5.1   Cervical dermatomes

(b) *Biochemical tests*. When there is serious bone disease the alkaline phosphatase will be raised. Bony secondaries of prostatic carcinoma will raise the acid phosphatase. In multiple myeloma there will be a myeloma band on the electrophoretic strip and Bence-Jones's protein in the urine.

(c) *Immunological tests*. If rheumatoid arthritis is

suspected then the rheumatoid factor will be present in the blood.

X-rays

Plain films

These are valuable for two reasons. Firstly they can be used to exclude serious disease such as secondary deposits. Secondly they can be used to find significant disruption of the spine. What they cannot do is tell whether degenerative change is responsible for symptoms. A full examination consists of four main views.

1 *Anteroposterior*, which allows problems such as secondary deposits and congenital abnormalities to be recognised.

2 and 3 *Lateral flexion and extension*, which shows disc degeneration, osteophytes and destruction of the vertebral bodies. More importantly it also shows if there is any significant slip at any level which may embarrass the spinal cord. A slip of up to 5 millimetres is acceptable at the C1–2 level (see Figure 5.2) but the leeway is much less lower down and slips at the C4–5 and C5–6 levels can cause quadriplegia.

4 *Open mouth*, to show the ondontoid. This is most important if a fracture is suspected.

Myelography

If compression of the spinal cord is suspected, then a myelogram should be performed to demonstrate the block in the free flow of contrast in the spinal canal. This investigation should not be undertaken unless everyone concerned is committed to proceed to surgery if a block is demonstrated.

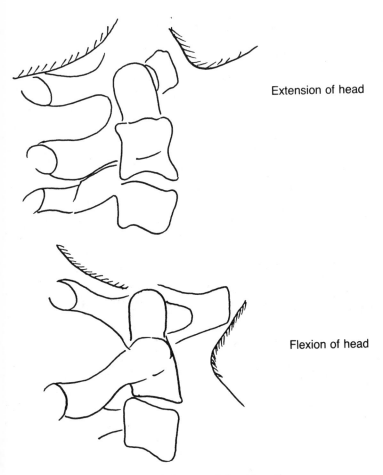

Extension of head

Flexion of head

Figure 5.2   Atlanto-axial subluxation

Bone scan

This is useful if there is any question of secondary deposits or infection in the neck. Changes are seen much earlier than with plain X-ray.

Specific Conditions

Rheumatoid arthritis (RA)

Neck involvement is a considerable problem in advanced RA. Many patients complain of pain but if bone erosion and softening of the ligaments becomes severe there is the danger of there being a subluxation at one or more levels with subsequent pressure on the spinal cord. Surprisingly this is far more likely to happen in the mid-cervical region than at the atlanto-axial level, even though the latter is more common. Sometimes the diagnosis is difficult to make clinically as these patients frequently have gross hallux valgus which makes assessment of the plantar reflexes impossible and such bad hand involvement that muscle strength is hard to assess. Warning should be taken if the patient complains of loss of feeling, sudden loss of strength, including going off the feet, and the diminution of pain in the peripheral joints.

If the problem is just one of pain then a cervical collar can be prescribed. These collars do not restrict neck movement significantly and therefore the most comfortable one is the best to use, usually a soft collar. If there is evidence of cord pressure surgery should be considered. If this is not possible or accepted then proper external fixation with a Minerva jacket or halo traction is the only way of ensuring adequate fixation.

Ankylosing spondylitis (AS)

In advanced AS neck involvement is common and may

be more disabling than lumbar disease. Once the patient can no longer turn his neck then important activities such as driving become difficult, if not impossible. The stiffness will proceed the ossification on X-ray and the neck must be encouraged to remain as supple as possible and in a good posture. Luckily spinal cord pressure is rare. If the neck does become very stiff tasks such as driving can be facilitated by the careful placement of mirrors.

Psoriatic arthritis (PSA)

The mutilating variety of PSA frequently attacks the neck, causing severe pain, and can lead to quadriplegia.

Juvenile chronic arthritis (JCA)

This group of disorders is discussed fully in Chapter 11. Suffice it to say here that neck pain is a frequent complaint in the polyarticular variety of the disease and to a lesser extent in the systemic and pauciarticular types.

Cervical spondylosis(CS)

Osteoarthritis in the spine is called spondylosis. If the cervical spine of anyone over the age of 40 is X-rayed there will be evidence of CS. The majority of people are symptom-free and thus finding CS on X-ray cannot be used to account for neck pain. Certainly large osteophytes can encroach on nerve roots and large bony outgrowths in some patients are responsible for cervical myelopathy. The majority of neck pain is due, however, to soft tissue problems rather than CS.

Cervical disc protrusions

These are fairly uncommon but a small protrusion may well cause considerable problems if there is already narrowing of canal or foramen by osteophyte formation. The onset is usually dramatic, with sudden pain in the neck and the onset of neurological signs. The patient will usually get better with rest alone as the disc shrivels up, but a careful watch needs to be kept on the patient. If the physical condition deteriorates, urgent surgical intervention may be necessary.

Ligamentous lesions

These are probably the most common cause of symptoms related to the neck. Precise diagnosis is difficult in the absence of adequate investigational methods. There will be no neurological signs but referred pain into the arm or up into the head is common. Treatment is usually successful with simple analgesics and physiotherapy.

Fibromyalgia

This condition is a syndrome consisting of three elements.

1 Ligamentous or degenerative neck pain.
2 Trigger spots (+/− palpable 'fibrositic nodules') and painful skin pinch.
3 Sleep disturbance.

The condition responds to small doses of sleep-inducing antidepressants and physiotherapy to the underlying musculoskeletal problem.

Trauma

The neck is often injured in sport, at work and in the motor car, where whiplash is frequent in rear-end collisions. Once the acute pain has subsided the majority will respond to simple physiotherapy.

Malignant disease

Five carcinomas regularly metastasise to bone: lung, breast, prostate, kidney and thyroid, and all may cause collapse of vertebrae in the neck. The collapse can be distinguished from that due to infection because in malignant disease the disc space will be preserved.

CHAPTER 6

PAIN IN THE BACK

Introduction

Back pain can almost be regarded as a part of the normal human condition. In part this relates to our upright posture and in part to the considerable demands that we place on our backs. The vast majority of episodes of back pain are self-limiting. This chapter deals with those causes of back pain that will result in a patient seeking medical advice.

The History

The history is crucial in the management of back pain as it acts as the screen for those very few patients that require further investigation. By careful questioning as outlined below a lot of time and money can be saved.

1 How long has the pain been present?
2 Is this the first episode or has it occurred before?
3 Where in the back is the pain?

4 Does the pain move anywhere?
5 Is there anything that makes the pain worse?
6 Is there anything that improves the pain?
7 Is the pain there all the time?
8 Does the pain disturb sleep?
9 Is there any limitation of back movement?
10 Is there any stiffness and, if so, when is it worst?
11 Was there any obvious precipitating cause?
12 Are any other joints involved?
13 Are there any paraesthesiae?
14 Is there any weakness?
15 Is there any sphincter disturbance?
16 Are there any systemic symptoms?
17 Is there a significant past history?
18 Is there a significant family history?
19 What is the patient's job?
20 What treatment has been tried, and has it been effective?

Among the possible aggravating causes are coughing, sneezing, straining at stool, and bending and lifting. The most important factor improving the pain is to differentiate between rest and activity. If better when resting the pain is likely to be due to degenerative change; if when active, inflammation.

Systemic problems to be on the lookout for include skin rash, inflamed eyes, urethral discharge or dysuria, and inflammatory bowel disease.

Similarly in the family history the presence of psoriasis, ulcerative colitis, Crohn's disease, and inflammatory eye disease is important, as well as a history of arthritis or back pain.

An occupational history is important as well as finding out if there is an outstanding compensation claim.

The Examination

This is frequently done badly. It is true that as most of the structures in the back are deep inside the body it is frequently difficult to localise the site of a lesion accurately. If properly done a lot of information can be obtained. The patient should be properly undressed. A full physical examination must be undertaken because so many diseases can give pain in the back. Certainly this routine must be followed in any patient with persistent or unusual symptoms. In women this will include examining the breasts and, on occasion, doing a pelvic examination. Men may well require a rectal examination.

The patient will need to be examined standing and lying. Wherever possible measurements should be taken to help with following the progress of the disease. The elements of the examination are given in Table 6.1.

Table 6.1 *Examination of the lumbar spine*

Physical sign	Site	Cause
Scoliosis	Lumbar or dorsal	Congenital
		Acute disc prolapse
		Spondylosis
Kyphosis	Lumbar or dorsal	Muscle weakness
		Ankylosing spondylitis
		Osteoporosis
		Malignant disease
Loss of range	Lumbar or dorsal	Infection
		Ankylosing spondylitis
		Acute disc prolapse
		Spondylosis
		Osteoporosis
	Straight leg raise	Disc prolapse
		Spondylosis
		Ligamentous pain
		Hip disease

Table 6.1 (cont.)   Examination of the lumbar spine

Physical sign	Site	Cause
Tenderness	Spine	Spondylosis
		Osteoporosis
		Malignant disease
		Infection
	Sacroiliac joint	Ankylosing spondylitis
		Reiter's syndrome
		Spondylosis
		Infection
	Paraspinal structures	Ligamentous lesions
		Spondylosis
		Infection
		Malignant disease
	Loins	Fibromyalgia
Pain on movement	Lumbar spine – all movements (not all need be involved)	Ankylosing spondylitis
		Disc prolapse
		Spondylosis
		Ligamentous disease
		Osteoporosis
		Infection
		Malignant disease
	Lumbar spine – extension	Facet joint osteoarthritis
	Straight leg raise	Disc prolapse
		Spondylosis
		Ligamentous disease
		Hip disease
	Femoral stretch	Disc prolapse
		Spondylosis
		Ligamentous disease
	Dorsal spine	Ankylosing spondylitis
		Osteoporosis
		Scheuermann's disease
		Malignant disease
		Infection
Weakness	Trunk	Dermatomyositis and polymyositis
		Muscular dystrophy
		Other neurological diseases
	Legs	Disc prolapse
		Cord lesions
		Peripheral neuritis
		Multiple sclerosis
		Other neurological diseases

Table 6.1 (cont.)   Examination of the lumbar spine

Physical sign	Site	Cause
Reflex and sensory changes	Legs	Disc prolapse Cord lesions Peripheral neuritis Multiple sclerosis Other neurological diseases

Abnormal postures of the lumbar spine may be due either to an acute muscle spasm protecting a painful lesion are to an anatomical abnormality. Hence the presence of pain and obvious muscle spasm should be sought.

With loss of range it is also important to decide if the loss of range is due to pain or anatomical abnormality. It is important to remember that the ability to touch the toes does not depend on lumbar spine movement but on having a good range in the hips, together with the absence of stretch on an irritated sciatic nerve. Lumbar flexion should therefore be measured by employing the Schober test (Figure 6.1) or by using a special goniometer. A less accurate method is to place the four fingers on the patient's lumbar spinous processes and get him to bend forwards and then back. The processes will be felt to move apart and then back together.

If ankylosing spondylitis is suspected a confirmatory test is to measure chest expansion. The patient places his hands behind the head and the tape measure placed around the chest at nipple level. A deep breath is taken and then full expiration. Although chest expansion varies with age and build, a finding of less than 5 centimetres in an adult is abnormal.

If there is nerve root pressure at the L4–5 or L5–S1 levels the straight leg raise (SLR) will be reduced. In

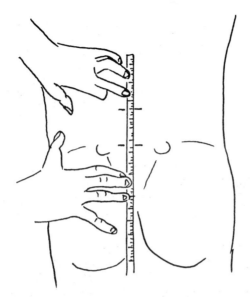

Figure 6.1   Schober test

acute disc prolapse only a few degrees will be possible
but as the patient improves, so will the raise. Lesser
degrees of restriction are seen with referred pain into
the leg from ligamentous or degenerative disease, but
there will be no neurological signs. SLR can be checked
in the hypersensitive or dishonest patient either by
flexing the knee and then flexing the hip or by getting
the patient to sit up (as in examining the back of the
chest) with the legs out straight. In the first test there
should be no pain and in the second the manoeuvre
should be impossible. SLR will be invalidated if there is
significant hip disease.

Tenderness of the sacroiliac joint can be tested in a
number of ways but all are unreliable. The patient can
be laid on his side and pressure exerted on the
up-facing hip. Direct pressure can be applied to each

joint. With the patient face-down pressure can be exerted on the sacrum.

Tenderness, with or without the presence of 'nodules', is typical of fibromyalgia.

It is most uncommon for there to be pain on all movements of the spine in degenerative or ligamentous pain. If all are painful then an inflammatory or other serious disorder must be actively excluded.

The various signs and symptoms related to nerve root pressure are given in Table 6.2 and Figure 6.2. Referred pain into the legs from the lumbar spine is common and produces symptoms in the territory of the dermatome related to the level at which the spine or paraspinal structures are being irritated. There will be the absence of neurological signs.

Table 6.2 *Lumbar root signs and symptoms*

Root	Area of pain	Muscle weakness	Jerk changes
L1	Upper lumbar area, groin and buttock	—	—
L2	Lower lumbar area, upper buttock and upper thigh	Psoas	—
L3	Front and inner aspect of thigh to knee	Quadriceps	Knee
L4	Outer thigh and calf to foot	Tibialis anterior, extensor hallucis longus	—
L5	Down back of leg to foot – 'classical sciatica'	Extensor hallucis longus, peronei, gluteus medius	Ankle

Investigation of Back Pain

Because so many disorders can present as back pain, including intra-abdominal disease, it is not practical to

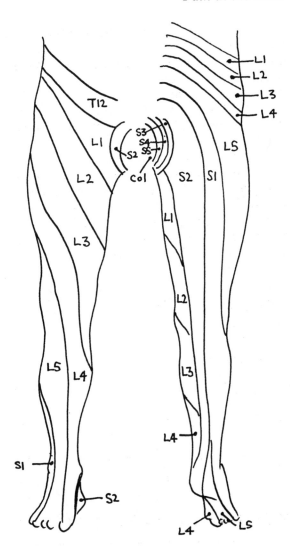

Figure 6.2 Lumbo-sacral dermatomes

list here the full range of tests that could conceivably be done in the investigation of back pain. However, those that are appropriate to the majority of patients presenting will be discussed.

Blood tests

(a) *Haemoglobin*. If an anaemia is found it is likely to for three reasons. The first is that it is the normochromic, normocytic anaemia of chronic inflammation in ankylosing spondylitis, although this is usually not particularly marked. The second reason is malignant disease, including disseminated carcinoma and multiple myeloma. Lastly it may be due to gastrointestinal bleeding associated with taking analgesics.

(b) *White cell count*. This may be raised in infections in the spine.

(c) *Sedimentation rate*. The ESR is probably the most helpful investigation in persistent back pain. Many of the most common painful conditions will not elevate the ESR, including disc prolapse, spondylosis, ligamentous disease and osteoporosis. If it is elevated, further tests are mandatory. By the same token other non-specific tests, such as the plasma viscosity and c-reactive protein, are of value as screening tests.

(d) *Alkaline phosphatase*. This will be elevated in conditions causing an increased turnover in bone. Modest elevation is seen in secondary deposits (especially from the prostate), infection and osteomalacia. Very high levels can be seen in Paget's disease of bone, even from a quite small focus, such as a single vertebra.

(e) *Acid phosphatase.* This is elevated in prostatic carcinoma and it is wise to ask for this test in any male patient who complains of persistent back pain. Performing a rectal examination may increase the level, and hence should be avoided prior to doing the test.

(f) *Electrophoretic strip.* Multiple myeloma will produce a discrete band, while an inflammatory pattern will be present in a wide range of systemic conditions.

Urine tests

Bence-Jones's protein will be detected in multiple myeloma.

X-rays

(a) *Plain films.* It is important to remember that past the age of 40 the vast majority of people will show evidence of degenerative change on plain films. Therefore the finding of spondylosis should not be taken as the cause of the back pain. The main use of the plain film is to exclude the possibility of more serious disease being present. If bone replacement is being looked for the best view is the posteroanterior view, which allows the pedicles to be examined, as they show erosion earliest. This view also allows such features as syndesmophytes, osteophytes, dense vertebrae due to Paget's disease, and congenital abnormalities to be identified.

Lateral views show osteoporosis, sepsis (which will involve the disc space), squaring of the vertebral bodies in early ankylosing spondylitis, secondary deposits, and osteophytes. This view will also show slipping of one vertebra on another (spondylolisthesis) and fractures in the pedicles (spondylolysis). It is usually not necessary to do oblique views to check on the possibility of spondylolysis.

The plain X-ray of the pelvis is the best method of making the diagnosis of ankylosing spondylitis as a good view of the sacroiliac joints is obtained and other features can be identified.

(b) *Contrast films.* Where lesions compressing the spinal canal or the nerve roots, while they run within the nerve sheaths, are suspected then contrast studies are of considerable value. The most popular study is the radiculogram, using water-soluble contrast which gives better definition than oil-based myelography. A radiculogram should not be contemplated unless there is a firm commitment to proceeding to surgery by all concerned if an operable lesion is shown. The study is most used to demonstrate a prolapsed intervertebral disc but can also show spinal stenosis and other space-occupying lesions in and around the spinal canal such as a neurofibromata or secondary deposit.

Some authorities advocate other contrast techniques such as discograms and ascending lumbar venography but they should be reserved for specialist centres.

(c) *Tomography.* Simple tomograms are useful for examining the structure of the bone, especially if there is the possibility of bone destruction. The much wider availability of computerised tomography has greatly enhanced the possibility of accurately making an anatomical diagnosis, but it is an expensive technique and should be reserved for the more obscure cases.

(d) *Bone scan.* This is often a 'best buy' in the investigation of prolonged back pain. It will show secondary deposits long before plain X-ray, as well as showing infection and areas of significant degenerative disease. It should be considered in any patient with a known cancer who presents at a later date with back pain.

(e) *Bone density*. It is now possible to measure bone density by a number of techniques and this is of considerable value in the management of osteoporosis.

Specific Conditions

Ankylosing spondylitis (AS)

This is a condition affecting about 1 in 200 people. Although it is most commonly recognised in men it does occur in women almost as often, but tends to be much milder and is also atypical with more peripheral disease. It is thus much less frequently diagnosed.

The history is usually one of low back pain that is at its worst first thing in the morning and after prolonged inactivity. It is improved by exercise and by taking non-steroidal drugs. There may be an associated iritis. Apart from the back disease the condition can also move to the neck and to peripheral joints. Tests for sacroilitis may or may not be present and the X-ray is a much better way of finding the changes. The first changes in the spine happen at the dorsolumbar junction. A full description is given in Chapter 2. If the hips are uninvolved the patient may well be able to touch his toes; hence the patient must be properly undressed to assess movement. Chest expansion is very frequently reduced.

Other seronegative arthropathies

The back problem associated with this group of disorders will be indistinguishable from AS and it is only the presence of the other features of the individual conditions that will make the diagnosis obvious. However, the sacroilitis is often asymmetrical on X-ray.

Prolapsed intervertebral disc (PID)

PID only represents about 10 per cent of cases of acute back pain but can be disabling and can on occasion be an emergency with acute retention of urine. The onset is usually sudden, with pain coming on when lifting and bending. There will be severe pain into the leg and examination will reveal the appropriate physical signs (see above). The plain X-ray will be normal as the disc space will not become reduced in size until 3 or 4 months after the nucleus pulposus has prolapsed, as the annulus will hold the bones apart for some time. The majority of acute PIDs will get better with rest and analgesics alone but in persistent cases, particularly if there is considerable muscle weakness, a period of bed rest in hospital is required. If the problem continues then radiculography and surgery should be actively considered. If the neurological signs are improving but pain remains a problem, a steroid epidural injection should be considered.

Central disc prolapses can give rise to cauda equina claudication, especially if the canal is narrowed congenitally or by osteophytes. In this syndrome there is pain and paraesthesiae, brought on by walking or other activity. The peripheral pulses will be present and there may be neurological signs. There is the risk of urinary retention and permanent weakness if not corrected.

Spondylosis

Osteoarthritis in the spine is called spondylosis. As has been stressed above, virtually all people over the age of 40 have evidence of spondylosis on X-ray but that does not mean that the symptoms being complained of are due to those appearances. None the less spondylosis clearly is implicated in the production of a lot of back pain, probably by direct pressure on soft tissues or by abnormally stressing them. In the lumbar spine osteophytes rarely encroach on the nerve roots, as they do in the neck. New bone formation can certainly embarrass an already stenosed canal. It should be noted, however, that the biggest osteophytes seen are in disseminated idiopathic skeletal hyperostosis (see below) and these virtually never give trouble. In the absence of neurological signs spondylosis should be treated as for ligamentous disease, with rest, analgesics, physiotheraphy and advice about using the back properly in future.

Spinal stenosis

The spinal canal can be narrowed congenitally or the condition can be acquired. The most common form of congenital narrowing is the trefoil configuration (see Figure 6.3). This will not necessarily give trouble until late life when disc degeneration and spondylosis may further encroach on the canal. In the normal canal, these two factors can cause the problem themselves, if severe enough.

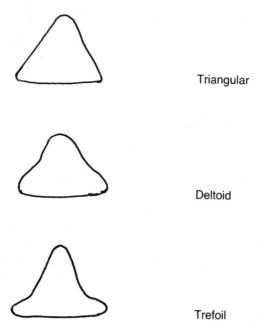

Triangular

Deltoid

Trefoil

Figure 6.3   Spinal canal cross-sections

Treatment is by surgical decompression.

Spondylolisthesis and spondylolysis

When there is slippage of one vertebra on another it is

called spondylolisthesis.In the majority of cases this is due to disc degeneration and osteoarthritis in the apophyseal joints allowing the normal anatomical relationships to become distorted. As such, this will not in itself cause symptoms. However, excessive stress on the pedicle will cause it to fracture – spondylolysis. This produces an unstable segment which is usually painful. If it is, then the segment will need stabilisation surgically.

Disseminated idiopathic skeletal hyperostosis (DISH)

This is a condition with a number of different names – Forrestier's disease and ankylosing hyperostosis. It produces the most spectacular osteophytes on X-ray, which may be confused with ankylosing spondylitis or severe spondylosis. Elsewhere in the skeleton there will be considerable bony spurs and ossification at tendon insertions. DISH is associated with diabetes. It is a common incidental finding in the elderly and rarely gives symptoms. It can be safely ignored in the vast majority of patients.

Scheuermann's disease

This is a form of osteochondritis occurring in the dorsal and upper lumbar regions of adolescents. It tends to lead to backache in schoolchildren as they start to study hard for examinations, where the constant bent posture may aggravate the condition. It is self-limiting but can lead to kyphosis in later life. The X-ray appearances can be quite startling with irregularity in the margins of the affected vertebrae and anterior wedging.

Ligamentous back pain

This term covers a group of disorders, often of indeterminate pathological cause, that form the bulk of problems seen in the low back. There are a large number of structures around the spine, including ligaments, muscles, blood vessels, discs and glands, as well as the bone and joints. The area is richly innervated and any irritation of these nerves will lead to pain. Acute trauma, continuous stress, and degeneration in and around the apophyseal joints all lead to such irritation. The pain felt is often referred into the buttock or down the leg, in the dermatome associated with the level being irritated. Fibromyalgia is frequently seen, with sleep disturbance and trigger areas in the back (see Chapter 5). The majority of patients will get better spontaneously but get repeated attacks. To prevent these relapses an important part of the treatment is to teach the patient back care. Other important features of treatment are rest and analgesics in the acute phase and then physiotherapy as the patient improves. Important among the effective techniques is strengthening of the anterior abdominal wall, Maitland's manipulation and hydrotherapy. Treatment should be undertaken by an experienced physiotherapist who is skilled in assessment and the various treatments available.

Occasionally local intra-lesional steroid injection helps. In patients with the fibromyalgia syndrome a small dose of a sleep-inducing antidepressant may be of value.

Osteoporosis

Osteoporosis is seen in post-menopausal women, patients on steroid therapy following immobility and in old age. It is a common cause of severe back pain in women. There may be generalised aching punctuated by episodes of severe pain due to pathological fracture of one or more vertebrae. It may, to a certain extent, be avoided by keeping the steroid dose as low as possible, maintaining physical activity in the elderly and giving hormone replacement therapy in menopausal women. If symptomatic osteoporosis has occurred, treatment will include analgesics, encouragement to remain active, reduction in steroid dosage and specific therapy. Specific therapy is controversial but in the woman with severe post-menopausal osteoporosis, calcium supplements, fluoride and hormone replacement therapy is indicated. In milder cases calcium supplements may be sufficient, even though the problem is related to the matrix of the bone and not the calcium balance. In some elderly people there may be coexistent osteomalacia and there is an argument for giving a single dose of vitamin D in very elderly patients with thinning of the bones.

Paget's disease of bone

Small deposits of Paget's are common in elderly people and should be remembered if the alkaline phosphatase is very raised or there is a single dense vertebra.

Malignant disease

Secondary carcinomas frequently go to bone, especially

lung, breast, prostate, thyroid and kidney. The other common malignancy seen is multiple myeloma. These diagnoses must be borne in mind when the patient complains of unremitting pain, weight loss, symptoms possibly associated with a primary site or a history of previous cancer.

Bone scan is usually the best investigation for secondary deposits but myeloma does not show up as a rule, and a blood and urine screen should be done if this diagnosis is suspected.

Infection

Although tuberculosis is much less common than it was, infection, either acute or chronic, is still encountered from time to time. No matter what the organism the cardinal feature to be aware of in the X-ray is involvement of the disc space, which is invariably spared in malignant disease. In tuberculosis a psoas abscess will show up on the posteroanterior film as a marked paraspinal shadow. The patient is likely to complain of unremitting pain, weight loss, general malaise, fevers and, often, night sweats. If a potential focus of infection is found it is important to obtain an accurate bacteriological diagnosis which usually means performing a biopsy. This can often be done by percutaneous wide-bore needle biopsy. If it is not possible to obtain adequate material for bacteriology then it is probably worth treating empirically with anti-tuberculous therapy.

CHAPTER 7

PAIN IN THE HIP

Introduction

Osteoarthritis of the hip is a major cause of pain and disability in middle age, and hip involvement in diseases such as rheumatoid arthritis and ankylosing spondylitis in younger people can make for considerable problems in mobility and sexual function. It is important to recognise hip pain because it is the joint *par excellence* that can be treated surgically.

The History

The most important aspect of taking the history in conditions associated with the hip is to remember that many patients are unaware of the location of the hip joint itself, and when they say that they have hip pain they are much more likely to mean that they have pain in the buttock or low back. Hip pain is usually felt in the groin, down the thigh, and in the knee. If a patient complains of knee pain it is essential to examine the hip, even if there appears to be a reason for the pain in the knee. Hip pain does not radiate below the knee.

As with other joints, various questions need to be answered in patients with hip-related pain.

1 How long has the pain been present?
2 Is this the first episode or has it occurred before?
3 Are both hips involved?
4 Does weight-bearing make the pain worse?
5 Is there pain at rest and especially at night?
6 Is there limitation of range?
7 Is there stiffness and, if so, when is it at its worst?
8 Are there any functional problems?
9 Are there any sexual problems?
10 Was there any obvious precipitating cause?
11 Are there any other joints (including the spine) involved?
12 Are there any systemic symptoms?
13 Is there a significant past history?
14 Is there a significant family history?
15 What treatment has been tried and has it been effective?

The nature of hip pain can be variable. Many patients complain of pain only with weight-bearing while others notice the most trouble with night pain.

Limitation of range may not be very obvious to the patient if there is good back and knee movement but sitting, particularly in confined spaces such as a car, is the most troublesome problem initially. However a fixed or limited hip may give considerable problems with personal hygiene, sexual activity and with simple tasks like putting on socks or cutting toenails. An enquiry about these last two activities frequently reveals the cause of the problem.

Stiffness is not only a feature of inflammatory

diseases such as rheumatoid arthritis but is also seen in osteoarthritis. In the latter condition stiffness tends to be short-lived but occurs after even short periods of rest.

The Examination

After a proper history has been obtained the hip can be examined. The patient needs to be adequately undressed and should be examined both lying and standing. It is impossible to examine the hip properly without lying the patient flat. In standing the Trendelenburg test (see below) can be performed and the gait can be assessed. In patients complaining of 'hip' pain it is important to examine the back, as this is likely to be the source of the pain. The main features to look for in the hip are given in Table 7.1.

Because the hip joint is very deep, swelling associated with the joint is most uncommon. If a swelling is present it is much more likely to be due to a hernia or enlarged lymph glands. Similarly tenderness around the joint is likely to be due to things other than arthritis, but tenderness may be present in acute arthritis.

Table 7.1 Examination of the hip

Physical sign	Site	Causes
Tenderness	Groin	Rheumatoid arthritis
		Other inflammatory arthritides
		Lymph glands
	Greater trochanter	Trochanteric bursitis
	Pubic ramus	Fracture
		Adductor strain

Table 7.1 (cont.)   Examination of the hip

Physical sign	Site	Causes
Pain on movement	Flexion only – knee extended	Sciatic nerve tension
	All movements (not all need be involved)	Rheumatoid arthritis
		Ankylosing spondylitis
		Other seronegative arthritides
		Osteoarthritis
		Paget's disease of bone
		Fracture
		Aseptic necrosis
		Infection
		Malignant disease
		Bleeding disorders
		Regional osteoporosis
Loss of range	Flexion only – knee extended	Sciatic nerve tension
	All movements (not all need be involved)	Rheumatoid arthritis
		Ankylosing spondylitis
		Other seronegative arthritides
		Osteoarthritis
		Paget's disease
		Fracture
		Aseptic necrosis
		Infection
		Bleeding disorders
Special tests	Leg length discrepancy	Osteoarthritis
		Fracture
		Aseptic necrosis
		Congenital dislocation
		Old infection
		Juvenile chronic arthritis
		Scoliosis
		Rickets
	Trendelenburg test	Osteoarthritis
		Rheumatoid arthritis
		Other inflammatory arthritides
		Congenital dislocation
	Trendelenburg gait	Osteoarthritis
		Congenital dislocation
		Inflammatory arthritis

Sciatic nerve stretch reduces the straight leg raise and directs attention to the back. The same is true if there are neurological signs.

Fixed flexion of the hip is measured by fixing the pelvis with one hand and then flexing the contralateral hip. If there is fixed flexion the leg being examined will rise from the couch (Figure 7.1).

In most inflammatory diseases and osteoarthritis the first movements to become painful and limited are internal rotation and abduction.

Leg length discrepancy is most important to detect. Apart from giving important information about the damage to the hip it may also explain back pain related to an abnormal pelvic tilt which accompanies hip disease, as well as being seen in other cases of shortened leg. Two measurements are made – the true and apparent lengths. The true length is measured from the anterior superior iliac spine, which can be felt in even the fattest patient, to the medial malleolus of the tibia. It is important to ensure that the patient is lying flat and is as straight as possible, with the knee extended. Apparent length, which measures pelvic tilt as a rule, is taken from a fixed central point, such as the xiphisternum, and measures to the medial malleolus. Again it is important to have the patient straight and flat.

The Trendelenburg test is used to identify a diseased hip. The patient is examined standing, from behind. He is asked to stand on one foot. If the hip is intact the pelvis on the opposite side will rise. If hip disease is present the pelvis will drop, due to weakness of the abductors.

The typical gait of hip disease is also called Trendelenburg. In this there is a lurch towards the side of the bad hip during the stance phase of walking.

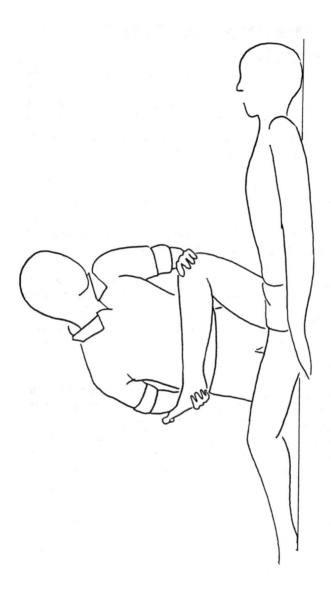

Figure 7.1   Testing for fixed flexion of the hip

The Investigation of the Painful Hip

If hip disease is discovered it is sensible to do screening tests for the causes of polyarthritis as detailed in Chapter 2. In this section only those tests applicable to the hip itself will be mentioned.

Blood tests

(a) *White cell count.* A neutrophilia may point to acute sepsis as the cause for sudden hip pain.

(b) *Sedimentation rate.* This acts as a useful screening test to differentiate degenerative from inflammatory disease. Very occasionally polymyalgia rheumatica (see Chapter 5) will present predominately with pain around the pelvis and a raised ESR may help to make the diagnosis.

(c) *Alkaline phosphatase.* Paget's disease of bone most commonly attacks the pelvis and femora and a very high alkaline phosphatase will be present. More modest elevations may be seen in rheumatoid arthritis (where it will be derived from the liver) and in bone destruction in infection and malignant disease.

(d) *Acid phosphatase.* Secondary prostatic carcinoma frequently attacks the pelvis and will be distinguished by this test.

(e) *Plasma electrophoresis.* This may reveal the discrete myeloma band.

(f) *Immunological tests*. The rheumatoid factor is a useful screen in patients presenting with a large joint arthritis rather than the more normal polyarthritis.

X-ray

(a) *Plain films*. The best view to take for the hip is a full anteroposterior pelvic film. Not only will this give information about the hip joint but it will show the other joint for comparison, the pelvic bones, including the pubic rami and symphysis, the sacroiliac joints and the lower lumbar vertebrae, all of which may be giving pain identified by the patient as 'hip' pain. Among the appearances that will be sought are narrowing of the joint space, deformity of the femoral head, osteophytes, erosions, protrusio acetabuli, abnormal calcification, fracture, both traumatic and pathological, bone destruction, and the remodelling of Paget's disease of bone.

(b) *Bone scan*. If it is uncertain that the pain is coming from minor degenerative changes the bone scan is of use. It will also show up inflammatory arthritis before there are much in the way of X-ray changes, pending aseptic necrosis, and the presence of secondary deposits. It may also show an osteoid osteoma which will be insignificant on plain X-ray.

Biopsy

If infection is suspected or there are unusual features, a biopsy may be considered. Normally a needle aspiration will be attempted first, under direct X-ray vision, but if this fails then the joint may need to be laid open for a bacteriological or histological specimen to be obtained.

Specific Conditions in the Hip and Surrounding Tissues

Rheumatoid arthritis (RA)

The hip is frequently involved in RA but may be overshadowed by small joint disease elsewhere. Typically the joint becomes narrowed, with pain on internal rotation. The femoral head then tends to become flat, and marked protrusio acetabuli will occur.

Hip involvement is most important in RA. It can seriously limit walking, make it difficult to get in and out of the car or a low seat, make sexual intercourse painful or impossible, and disturb sleep. Joint replacement should always be considered but it must be remembered that many other joints may be affected in the leg which may make a successful outcome much less certain.

Ankylosing spondylitis (AS)

Hip involvement is so common in AS that the joint may be regarded as a central joint in this disease. It is much more likely to be hip disease causing limitation in touching the toes than the back. Because of the enthesopathic inflammation seen in AS there may be pain and tenderness along the pubic ramus and over the greater trochanter.

Other seronegative arthropathies

Both Reiter's syndrome and psoriatic arthritis can attack the hip joints, causing considerable pain and disability.

Osteoarthritis (OA)

This is one of the most common problems in later life and costs considerable sums to treat. It occurs more commonly in people with evidence of generalised nodal osteoarthritis, the hallmark of which is the Heberden's node. The onset is usually gradual, with pain on walking and performing certain activities like cutting the toenails. The pain will be felt in the groin, down the front of the thigh and into the knee. Often the pain is only felt in the knee, which can be confusing for the patient and doctor alike. Night pain is frequent and can be debilitating. Immobility stiffness will be present, with a few paces being necessary to get the joint going.

The X-rays initially will show some loss of joint space and then osteophytes will appear, particularly as a fringe around the head of the femur. Sclerosis and subchondral cysts may be visible. Eventually the joint may become totally disrupted.

In the initial phase a number of simple measures can be undertaken. Weight reduction will reduce the load on the hip, as will using a walking stick in the contralateral hand. Muscle strengthening exercises and Maitland's peripheral mobilisations can be undertaken by the physiotherapist. Simple analgesics or non-steroidal anti-inflammatory drugs are beneficial. If simple measures fail then surgical replacement should be sought. This is a good operation with a high success rate, allowing an almost total return to normal life in most patients. Occasionally a patient is deemed not fit for operation or refuses one, in which case intra-articular steroid injections, done under direct X-ray vision, may be helpful.

Aseptic necrosis

The blood supply to the head of the femur is parlous and may fail for a number of reasons including fracture of the femoral neck, rheumatoid arthritis, systemic lupus erythematosus, caisson disease, sickle cell disease, and liver disease. It can also complicate high-dose steroid therapy but the evidence that it complicates the ingestion of analgesics is poor.

Typically the X-ray shows a rapid increase in density of the femoral head, then an equally rapid flattening and finally total destruction.

The only long-term solution to this problem is hip replacement.

Calcium pyrophosphate deposition disease (CPPD)

CPPD is frequently seen in the hip joint and gives rise to accelerated OA. Once the joint is worn away the calcification in the joint will disappear but may well be spotted in the other hip or the pubic symphysis if a full

pelvic X-ray has been taken.
Treatment is symptomatic, as for OA.

Apatite deposition

Although less common than painful arc syndrome a similar picture can be seen around the hip, with calcification visible in the trochanteric bursa. This produces pain on abducting the hip and is one of the causes of trochanteric bursitis (see below). It usually responds to a steroid injection.

Transient osteoporosis

This is a mysterious condition in which there is fairly rapid onset of osteoporosis in the femoral head. The hip remains painful for some time and then there is complete resolution. It occurs mainly in young men and affects either hip. It may occur during pregnancy in women, and then usually affects the left hip! This condition may be related to 'observation hip' seen in children where the hip becomes painful for several weeks or months but no radiological signs are found nor any systemic upset. Resolution is spontaneous and full.

Congenital dislocation of the hip (CDH)

This condition is an important cause of disability if it is not recognised. CDH occurs more frequently in females and in the white races more than blacks. It is due to a poorly developed acetabulum. All newborn babies should have their hips examined by abducting and adducting the joints and feeling for the characteristic click.

Treatment in the first few weeks of life is to splint the legs in abduction, which leads to proper development of the hips. If not discovered until later life, considerable leg shortening is likely with a Trendelenburg gait. Osteoarthritis is almost inevitable, with considerable pain, and total hip replacement is the only way to help the patient. This, however, is technically difficult because of the shallow acetabulum.

Perthe's disease

This is a form of juvenile osteochondritis, mainly affecting young boys. The hip is painful and X-ray shows a typical appearance of early aseptic necrosis, with flattening of the femoral head. Pressure needs to be taken off the head during the active phase, either by splintage or osteotomy. The head slowly revascularises over 3 or 4 years and if the joint has not been too badly damaged will give no further trouble, but OA is frequently seen later.

Short leg syndrome

If one leg is shorter than the other, for whatever reason, abnormal stresses are placed on the back and the knee. There is likely to be low back pain or pain in the knee. If the leg lengths are equilibrated by building up the shoe or by surgical correction the pain is usually relieved.

Paget's disease of bone

The pelvis and femur are frequent sites for Paget's disease. The affected bone is extensively remodelled, with thickening and coarse trabeculation. The bone is weaker than normal bone. The alkaline phosphatase is usually grossly elevated. The most common complaint is of deep unremitting pain but this is variable. If the hip joint is involved osteoarthritis will occur. Pathological fractures are seen and, rarely, sacromatous change.

Treatment is a little controversial. Simple analgesics may be sufficient but, if not, some form of specific therapy may be necessary. The most popular form is calcitonin but diphosphonates and mithramycin are used. The treatment is expensive and of variable outcome. Where there is secondary OA hip, hip replacement is very successful and remarkably trouble-free.

Osteoid osteoma

This tiny tumour is often found in the femur, producing quite severe, boring pain. It may be very difficult to identify on plain X-ray but a bone scan may be helpful in picking up the lesion.

The pain is usually abolished by aspirin but definitive treatment is by excision of the lesion.

Trochanteric bursitis

This is an underdiagnosed problem. It causes pain on

the outer aspect of the thigh over the greater trochanter with tenderness on pressure on the trochanter or just above it. Most arise spontaneously and may represent a form of enthesopathy. Some are associated with apatite deposition while others complicate inflammatory joint disease.

Treatment is by steroid injection, which is usually curative.

CHAPTER 8

PAIN IN THE KNEE

Introduction

The knee is an important weight-bearing and mobility joint. It is involved in many disease processes. It is also the joint that is the easiest to examine internally, by arthrography, joint aspiration, blind biopsy and arthroscopy. It should be remembered that it is not one joint but two: the tibiofemoral and the patellofemoral. The superior tibiofibular joint is also in close proximity. It is also important to remember that pain in the knee may well be referred, usually from the hip but also from the back, and both need to be examined in knee pain.

The History

A careful history will go a long way towards finding the cause of pain in the knee. The following questions need to be asked.

1   How long has the pain been present?
2   Is this the first episode or has it occurred before?
3   Are both knees involved?
4   Is the pain there only on weight-bearing or does it occur at rest?
5   Does the pain disturb sleep?
6   Is there limitation of movement or deformity?
7   Has there been any 'locking'?
8   Has there been any swelling?
9   Is there any stiffness and, if so, when is at its worst?
10   Is the knee unstable?
11   Are there any other joints involved?
12   Are there any paraesthesiae?
13   Is there any weakness?
14   Are there any systemic symptoms?
15   Is there a significant past history?
16   Is there a significant family history?
17   What treatment has been tried and, if any, has it been effective?

Locking is a symptom of internal derangement of the knee, usually a torn cartilage. The story is one of a twisting injury followed by the sudden sticking in one position, usually flexed. In severe cases there is considerable pain and the knee will not straighten – an orthopaedic emergency. In milder cases the knee will straighten but recurrence is likely.

Swelling may occur behind the knee and calf, as well as in front of the joint.

The Examination

It is important to emphasise that the examination of

Table 8.1   Examination of the knee

Physical sign	Site	Causes
Swelling		
soft tissue	Anterior knee	Rheumatoid arthritis
		Ankylosing spondylitis
		Other seronegative arthritides
		Pigmented villonodular synovitis
	Calf	Ruptured knee joint
bony	Generalised	Osteoarthritis
		Old rheumatoid
		Neuropathic joint
		Pyrophosphate deposition disease
effusion	Knee	Rheumatoid arthritis
		Ankylosing spondylitis
		Other seronegative arthritides
		Systemic lupus erythematosus
		Osteoarthritis
		Gout
		Pyrophosphate deposition disease
		Infection
		Bleeding disorders
		Pigmented villonodular synovitis
Wasting	Quadriceps	Any painful knee condition
		Lower motor neurone lesions
Tenderness	Knee	Rheumatoid arthritis
		Other inflammatory arthritis
		Gout
		Pyrophosphate deposition disease
		Rheumatic fever
		Infection
		Bleeding disorders
	Medial ligament	Osteoarthritis
		Hypermobility syndrome
	Tibial tubercle	Osgood–Schlatter disease

Table 8.1 (cont.) **Examination of the knee**

Physical sign	Site	Causes
Pain on movement	Flexion	Rheumatoid arthritis
		Ankylosing spondylitis
		Psoriatic arthritis
		Reiter's syndrome
		Colitic arthritis
		Systemic lupus erythematosus
		Osteoarthritis
		Gout
		Pyrophosphate deposition disease
		Chondromalacia patellae
		Trauma
		Infection
		Bleeding disorders
		Hypertrophic pulmonary osteoarthropathy
		Sarcoid
		Prepatellar bursitis
	Infrapatellar	Osteoarthritis
		Chondromalacia patellae
	Hip movements	Referred pain from hip
Loss of range	Flexion	Rheumatoid arthritis
		Ankylosing spondylitis
		Other seronegative arthritides
		Systemic lupus erythematosus
		Osteoarthritis
		Gout
		Pyrophosphate deposition disease
		Infection
		Bleeding disorder
		Prepatellar bursitis
		Trauma
		Neuropathic joint
		Pigmented villonodular synovitis
Deformity	Knee	Rheumatoid arthritis
		Osteoarthritis
		Pyrophosphate deposition disease
		Trauma
		Neuropathic joint
		Bleeding disorders

the knee is not complete without a full assessment of the hip as referred pain in the knee may be the only symptom of which the patient will complain. The details of the examination are given in Table 8.1.

Experience will allow the doctor to differentiate between the different types of swelling. There are a variety of ways for testing for effusion. If there is a large one a patella tap will be present (see Figure 8.1). A small amount of fluid is detected by using the 'wipe' sign (see Figure 8.2). If there is a large, tense effusion neither sign will be positive but this is usually obvious.

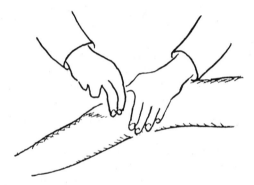

Figure 8.1   Patella tap

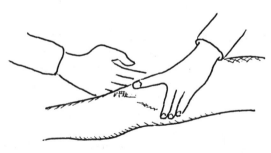

Figure 8.2   Wipe sign

If an effusion is present there is always the risk of the joint rupturing. This will produce a sudden pain in the calf, followed by calf swelling. In itself it is not serious but can be confused with deep vein thrombosis. Homans's sign will be positive and the calf tender, but the history of previous joint disease plus the sudden onset coupled with a positive arthrogram should make the diagnosis obvious.

Wasting of the quadriceps muscles occurs rapidly in any painful condition of the knee. This is most obvious in the trained athlete but may not be so in the obese elderly person. Measuring the circumference of the muscle is of some help but is quite inaccurate and is best reserved for following the progress of an individual undergoing treatment.

An inflammatory condition will cause tenderness in the joint generally, but the acute point tenderness felt on the medial side of the tibia at the insertion of the medial ligament is typical of patients with unstable osteoarthritic or hypermobile knees who place abnormal strains on the ligament.

Pain behind the patella is brought out by getting the patient to forcibly extend the knee down onto the couch while stabilising the top of the patella with the edge of the examiner's hand. If there is roughening of the back of the patella, this manoeuvre will be extremely painful.

The stability of the joint needs to be tested. The knee can be unstable laterally or in the anteroposterior direction. The former is tested by flexing the knee by about 20 degrees. This eliminates the effects of the locking that occurs in the final 5 degrees or so of extension, as well as any stability being offered by the quadriceps. The examiner then grasps the thigh in the left hand and attempts to rock the tibia in a pendular fashion sideways with the right hand. AP stability is sought by the draw sign. The patient flexes the knee to 90 degrees and the foot is stabilised by the examiner either sitting on it or resting the right elbow on it. The examiner then links his hands behind the upper end of the tibia and gently exerts pressure towards himself. If there is any cruciate instability the tibia will move forward on the femur.

If a torn cartilage is suspected McMurray's test should be undertaken. In this the hip and knee are flexed. The hip is then externally rotated and abducted and a further external rotational force applied to the ankle and the knee extended. The knee is flexed again and an internal rotatory force applied to the ankle and the knee extended again. The hip and knee are then flexed again and the two manoeuvres repeated with the hip adducted and internally rotated. The examiner's free hand is placed on the knee to feel for 'clicks' and the patient's face watched to see if pain is produced in any of the four positions.

Investigating the Knee

The majority of this section will concentrate on diagnostic procedures that are of special relevance to the knee. Screening tests and tests for specific systemic forms of arthritis are described in Chapter 2.

X-ray

(a) *Plain films.* The standard views are the anteroposterior and the lateral. These give considerable information (see Table 8.2). An additional film that is always worth taking when cartilage damage is expected is the

Table 8.2   X-ray changes in the knee

Lesion	Cause
Osteopenia	Osteomalacia
	Osteoporosis, especially disuse
	Algodystrophy
	Inflammatory arthritis
Change in bone structure	Paget's disease of bone
	Malignant disease
	Hyperparathyroidism
Sclerosis	Osteoarthritis
	Osteochondritis dissecans
New bone	Osteoarthritis
Erosions	Rheumatoid arthritis
	Seronegative arthritis
	Crystal deposition disease
	Sepsis
	Bleeding disorders
Loss of joint space	Osteoarthritis
	Rheumatoid arthritis
	Seronegative arthritis
	Crystal deposition disease
	Sepsis
	Bleeding disorders
Calcification	Pyrophosphate deposition disease
Deformity	Osteoarthritis
	Rheumatoid arthritis
	Seronegative arthritis
	Crystal deposition disease
	Bleeding disorders
	Neuropathic joints
	Trauma
	Juvenile chronic arthritis
Periosteal reaction	Hypertrophic pulmonary
	osteoarthropathy
	Juvenile chronic arthritis
	Osteomyelitis
	Hyperparathyroidism
	Bleeding disorders
	Thyroid acropachy

AP weight-bearing film. This will show acurately the amount of joint space narrowing. Another useful view is the skyline view, which allows examination of the back of the patella, particularly useful in looking for chondromalacia patellae. Unless there is very good reason it is as well to X-ray both knees, no matter which views are being taken.

(b) *Contrast films*. The arthrogram is used to look for synovial leaks into the calf. Joint rupture can be confused with deep vein thrombosis and this is therefore an important diagnosis to make. A needle is inserted into the joint and any fluid removed for analysis (see below). A small quantity of contrast medium is injected and the patient asked to walk around for a few minutes. If there is a significant synovial fluid leak contrast will be seen tracking down into the calf. This investigation should be done as soon as possible after the onset of symptoms as the defect tends to heal over within 2 days or so.

Fluid analysis

No joint is more accessible than the knee. Often effusions are of considerable volume and there are three routes for inserting a needle. The technique can be undertaken in the clinic or in the patient's home. It is not necessary to use a full sterile technique, a no-touch being quite safe. The easiest method is to have the patient sitting up on the couch with both legs extended. It is important that the patient is comfortable and that he knows what is happening. The skin is cleaned with a suitable spirit-based preparation and allowed to dry, to make the injection more comfortable. If the knee is to be injected after the aspiration, the injection can be drawn up at this time (see Chapter 12). Using a wide-bore needle the joint is punctured from the medial side, just below the lower edge and at the mid-point of the patella, at an angle of 45 degrees (see Figure 8.3). The needle will be felt going through the joint capsule into the joint cavity and fluid can then be withdrawn. It is best to aspirate to dryness for therapeutic purposes.

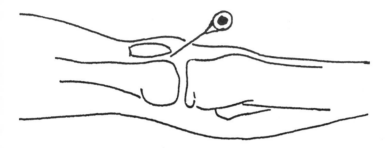

Figure 8.3   Site of injection of the knee

The other two routes are laterally, again at the mid-point of the patella, and through the infrapatellar tendon. In this approach the knee is flexed to 90 degrees and the joint entered by placing the needle through the tendon parallel to the tibial plateau. This is the most certain method of entering the joint and is perhaps best reserved for the small effusion or the very obese patient where problems may exist about defining the anatomy.

The typical findings of the aspirated fluid in the various conditions encountered are given in Table 8.3.

Table 8.3   *The analysis of joint fluid*

Disease	Appearance	Viscosity	White cells	Neutrophils (%)	Special features
'Normal'	Transparent, clear	High	Very low	<25	Nil
Degenerative	Transparent, yellow	High	Very low	<25	Nil
Inflammatory arthritis	Cloudy, yellow	Low	5000+ per cm^3	>50	Inflammatory cells
Crystal deposition disease	Cloudy	Low	5000+ per cm^3	>50	Crystals
Sepsis	Frank pus	Variable	50,000+ per cm^3	>90	Positive culture

Normally once the joint has been aspirated it will be injected with a steroid (see Chapter 12).

Biopsy

Again, because the knee is accessible, it is fairly easy to obtain tissue for histological examination. Three methods are available. The simplest is blind biopsy using a percutaneous needle. The advantages of this are that the equipment is cheap, the procedure can be performed in the clinic (in selected patients) and is easily learnt. The major disadvantage is that because pathological changes may be patchy in the synovium, the specimen may not be representative of the joint as a whole. Other disadvantages are that it is not always possible to be certain that synovium has been obtained, and the specimens are usually very small and distorted, which makes examination by the pathologist difficult.

Much better specimens may be obtained at arthroscopy. The exact site of biopsy can be chosen and multiple specimens obtained if a more representative picture is required. The technique is described in more detail below. Clearly the disadvantages are the cost of the equipment and the need for a skilled operator to use it.

The last method is open biopsy. This has become virtually obsolete with the advent of the arthroscope but may still be considered in difficult cases, especially where infection is strongly suspected and there is a need to obtain good material for bacteriological as well as histological examination, tuberculosis being the major indication. It should be avoided at all costs in children, as loss of range is almost inevitable.

This is not the place to itemise all the findings that the pathologist may see. However, it is worth pointing out that the number of different responses that the synovium can make is strictly limited and, unless a very specific appearance is seen, such as a typical rheumatoid nodule or acid-fast bacilli, the usual finding is of non-specific changes. The experienced pathologist can still make many useful comments under these circumstances and a biopsy is worth obtaining.

Arthroscopy

This is an extremely useful diagnostic tool which is increasingly being used for treatment as well. Essentially the arthroscope is a rigid telescope which allows the interior of the joint to be inspected. Normally there is a channel to allow biopsy forceps or other operative instruments to be inserted into the joint. Alternatively these can be inserted through a second incision. Normally the joint is inflated with saline to allow the best possible view.

It is possible to inspect the synovium, the joint surfaces and the menisci. Most of the joint can be examined with the exception of the most posterior portion. Among the abnormalities that can be seen are erosion in cartilage, synovial proliferation, torn menisci, crystals in the deposition diseases, loose bodies and the specific appearances of such diseases as villonodular synovitis. Biopsy sites can be chosen. By using the operating instrument torn menisci can be definitively treated without having to resort to arthrotomy.

Specific Conditions in the Knee

Rheumatoid arthritis (RA)

Although usually presenting as a small joint polyarthritis, the knee is a frequent site of monarticular onset. It may be several months before the polyarticular nature of the condition becomes obvious.

In established disease the knee is a target joint. RA will attack any joint that is being used regularly, particularly for weight-bearing. It is common for the joint to be damaged by the hydrostatic pressures being generated by large effusions. Synovial leaks are common. There is a distinct tendency for one or other of the tibial plateaux to collapse (usually the lateral). The effect is to produce a marked valgus or varus knee that rapidly gets worse as the centre of gravity moves outside the line of the leg, producing a bowstring effect. Large cysts, geodes, may form under the joint surfaces which can suddenly collapse or make surgical reconstruction extremely difficult. As mentioned, effusions are frequent in RA but some patients produce exuberant synovium. This (a) makes aspiration difficult as the fronds tend to block the needle and (b) makes steroid injection less successful than it might otherwise be. Another complication is the formation of fibrinous loose bodies, so-called melon-seed bodies. These again may block the needle on attempted aspiration. Effusions should be aspirated and the joint then injected with steroids. It is safe to do this up to three or four times in a 12-month period. If there is massive synovial proliferation a surgical synovectomy may still be worth considering. Radioactive synovectomy has not stood up well to careful clinical trial. If a lot of melon-seeds are being produced, washing the joint out may be beneficial. This is often done at the time of arthroscopy.

Quadriceps muscle wasting is almost inevitable. This tends to make the knee less stable and to lead to further joint damage. It is important to get the physiotherapist to supervise active quadriceps exercises.

In the badly damaged knee a number of surgical approaches are worth considering. Osteotomy may well help to re-align a leg that is going into varus or valgus. Knee replacement is now a successful operation as long as the prosthesis chosen matches the patient and the demands he will place on the new knee. Arthrodesis still remains a good operation for a selected group of patients where the aim is to produce a pain-free, stable leg.

Ankylosing spondylitis (AS)

If the AS patient is going to get peripheral arthritis, then the knee will usually be involved. The synovitis is clinically identical to that of RA, and histologically as well, apart from the absence of nodule formation. However, there is a tendency for the late stage to be bony ankylosis rather than the disorganisation seen in RA. Women tend to have more knee disease than men.

Treatment is as for RA.

Reiter's syndrome

Because Reiter's syndrome tends to affect lower limbs more than elsewhere, the knee is frequently troublesome. Recurrent effusions, night pain and difficulty walking may all bring the sufferer to the doctor. The patient with a painful knee should have a careful enquiry about previous diarrhoea, urethral discharge, red eye, and skin and mucosal lesions.

The knee can be treated by steroid injection and quadriceps exercises, as well as non-steroidal anti-inflammatory drugs, while recurrence is hopefully prevented by avoiding further non-specific urethritis or dysentery.

Colitic arthritis

The knee is the main target joint for the peripheral form of colitic arthritis. It is unusual for it to precede the colitis, so the diagnosis should not present problems. There is a marked tendency for the synovitis in the knee to come and go with the activity of the disease so that, apart from local measures, aggressive treatment of the colitis will settle the arthritis down. Colectomy should produce full remission of the arthritis.

Juvenile chronic arthritis (JCA)

Arthritis in children is described in detail in Chapter 11. The knee is frequently involved in JCA, particularly in the pauci-articular variety, in which it may be the only joint involved. It is essential to recognise it as there is the distinct possibility of blindness. There is usually an effusion and some soft tissue swelling. The joint is warm and there will be a distinct loss of function, most noticeable in young children who may go off their feet. Children are even more likely than adults to assume a position of comfort, and a fixed flexion deformity can rapidly develop.

Treatment is by analgesics and physiotherapy, which consists of passive straightening, splinting and active quadriceps exercises. Aspiration and steroid injection has now been shown to be safe, but may need to be done under sedation or anaesthetic.

Osteoarthritis (OA)

OA knee is extremely common. It is more likely to occur in patients with the generalised form of the disease, marked by Heberden's nodes, and in patients with previous knee injury, especially after surgery for torn meniscus. It is likely to be aggravated by obesity and arthritis in the hip or foot. It should also be remembered that hip disease may present as knee pain. OA can occur in the knee joint proper and in the patellofemoral joint. The complaint in either site is usually of pain on weight-bearing and immobility stiffness which makes the first few steps after sitting agony. Swelling may be noted and some patients will complain of a tender spot on the medial aspect of the knee. Some patients get night pain but this is less common than in OA hip.

Examination will often reveal OA in the hands, or an operation scar around the knee. There is likely to be an effusion present, which can be substantial. Bony swelling may also be felt and in the later stages there may be a valgus or varus deformity as the knee collapses. If the patellofemoral joint is involved there will be pain on forced extension of the knee (see above). There is frequently lateral instability of the joint and the insertion of the medial ligament will be painful. This is most frequently seen in obese women.

Treatment in the early stages can be satisfactorily achieved with weight loss, vigorous quadriceps exercises, non-steroidal anti-inflammatory drugs, and a walking stick, used in the opposite hand to the painful side. If an effusion is present, this should be aspirated and steroid injected. Occasionally, in later stages, a caliper can help but surgery may be required. Osteotomy may help to re-align the valgus or varus joint. Knee replacement is worth considering, while arthrodesis still has a limited place. Patellectomy should be avoided at all costs as the results are so poor.

Hypermobility syndrome

The amount of joint laxity experienced by a person depends, in the main, on the chemical structure of the collagen, which is an inherited factor. Some people have very 'loose' collagen leading to excessive joint laxity. A tiny minority suffer from a definite clinical condition, such as Marfan's syndrome. Most hypermobile people are very supple and do well at athletic activities. They may notice that their joints are loose ('double-jointed') and that their jaws 'click'. They can usually get their hands flat on the floor when asked to touch their toes and frequently their digits will be long and thin such that, when viewed from the dorsal side, the thumb can be placed across the palm and the tip appear beyond the medial border of the hand.

The importance of the condition is that many joints, but particularly the knee, are exposed to multiple minor injuries just in everyday activities. Knee pain and even effusion can occur. If steps are not taken to control the laxity OA can occur. Treatment is to undertake, on a regular basis, vigorous quadriceps exercises to 'take up the slack'. These patients should be encouraged to take regular exercise and to avoid muscle wasting at all costs.

Gout

Gout frequently attacks the knee producing intense pain, a large effusion, and the inability to walk. Aspiration of the joint helps both the diagnosis and the treatment. Urate crystals will be seen under the polarising light microscope. Removing the fluid and injecting with steroid will produce relief extremely rapidly.

Calcium pyrophosphate deposition disease (CPPD)

Ninety-eight per cent of patients with CPPD will have evidence of chondrocalcinosis articularis, both in the menisci and in the hyaline cartilage. It is also a major site for arthritis in CPPD. This can either be in the form of acute 'pseudogout' or chronic disease, leading to accelerated OA. In pseudogout there is an attack of acute arthritis of considerable intensity but, when the joint fluid is examined, it is found to contain pyrophosphate crystals. Treatment is with aspiration, injection and quadriceps exercises. The attacks are likely to be repetitive and will eventually lead to the chronic form. In this there is usually a chronic effusion, with pain on walking and immobility stiffness. Accelerated OA is the frequent end-point. Pyrophosphate crystals often will not be identified in the fluid in the chronic phase but can be seen on histological material. In the late stage the treatment is as for OA.

Infection

Any swollen joint may be infected. If an effusion is present it needs to be aspirated and sent for culture, even if there is known to be a pre-existing arthritis. Secondary infection in RA, for instance, is common and may be fatal if unrecognised and not treated. Sepsis is also common if there is an endoprosthesis present. If this is suspected a gallium bone scan is a helpful test.

Practically any organism can cause septic arthritis but this is not the place to list all the possibilities. One infection that is worth mentioning, however, is gonococcal arthritis which frequently affects the knee. It is surprisingly uncommon in Britain. There is usually a story of a sexual contact, followed by urethritis, a sparse skin rash, and then the arthritis. In women the urethritis might well go unnoticed and there may be denial of sexual contact. The rash may only be obvious on very close inspection. It tends to be found on the limbs, including the fingers, with a dark, even necrotic, centre. The joint involvement is an acute synovitis. It is usually possible to aspirate fluid from the knee if it is involved. In some cases the organism will be grown from the fluid but in the majority it will not be. This is because the majority of cases are in fact reactive arthritis rather than direct infection (cf. rheumatic fever and Reiter's syndrome). Diagnosis is made by blood culture, growing the organism from the skin lesions and by obtaining positive cultures from urethral, vaginal, rectal or throat swabs. The gonococcal fixation test is far too unreliable to be used diagnostically.

Bleeding disorders

Haemophilia and Christmas disease frequently present with haemarthrosis and again, it is the knee which is the most commonly involved joint. It is the repeated haemarthrosis and the consequent degeneration of the joint that represents the major cause of disability in this group of disorders. Most patients are aware of their condition and will present early with the onset of painful swelling of the joint. A effusion will be detected, which if it has been present for any length of time, tends to feel a little thicker than usual. Pain is intense and loss of function marked. Treatment is with the appropriate replacement blood factor and local treatment to the joint. There is some controversy about this. Elevation and the application of ice is helpful but joint aspiration is not favoured by all authors. However, if there is a large effusion then once the blood factor has been given, aspiration is safe and may prevent long-term damage to the joint.

Hypertrophic pulmonary osteoathropathy (HPOA)

HPOA is frequently identified on X-rays of the knee, either as several layers of periosteal reaction – onion skin, or as small raised nodules – candle wax. The knees are frequently painful. If these appearances are found a full search for the underlying cause must be undertaken.

Neuropathic joints

Any condition that produces a profound sensory neuropathy can lead to gross degeneration in a joint. This will frequently be the knee. The joint will be bizarrely deformed and often grossly unstable. Just because the underlying cause is denervation it does not mean that the joint will be pain-free. The classical cause is syphilis but it can be seen in diabetes (the feet), syringomyelia (the shoulder), or a variety of much rarer neurological conditions.

Sarcoid

The knee is often the site of sarcoid arthritis, especially if there is erythema nodosum. The ankles will also be involved. Synovial biopsy may reveal non-caseating granulomas. Chest X-ray will often show hilar lymphadenopathy.

Pigmented villonodular synovitis

This is a rare condition which can be regarded as a

locally invasive tumour. It occurs most frequently in the knee but may be seen in other joints. The joint is swollen, hot, tender and limited. Aspiration of an effusion, if one is present, will reveal serosanguineous fluid. The biopsy is characteristic with synovial proliferation, with increased vascularity, fibrosis, lymphocytes, giant cells, lipid containing macrophages, iron deposition and areas of haemorrhage. The treatment is synovectomy, which must be as complete as possible as recurrence is likely.

Chondromalacia patellae

This is a painful condition in which there is fibrillation of the cartilage of the patella. The cause is unknown. The pain can be reproduced by attempting forced extension of the knee against resistance (see above). The condition can be diagnosed by doing a skyline X-ray of the knee, which will reveal the fissures in the patella.

It frequently attacks young people and treatment is not easy. Quadriceps exercises sometimes help. Analgesics and non-steroidal agents give temporary relief. Patellectomy is a diastrous operation, frequently leading to a stiff knee or accelerated OA. If surgery is contemplated, the best available is to re-align the patellar tendon, which seems to take the strain off the articular surfaces.

Osgood–Schlatter disease

This is an osteochondritis of the tibial tubercle. It occurs in males, as a rule, between 10 and 16 years old.

About half the patients have bilateral disease. The tibial tubercle is very tender and X-ray will show irregularity of the tubercle. It resolves spontaneously.

Osteochondritis dissecans

This is a form of localised aseptic necrosis. There is an area of bone death leading to a small fragment becoming detached. There is considerable pain and there is likely to be locking. Surgery is usually required.

Torn meniscus

This is a common sporting injury. Typically there will be locking. Large lesions which come on rapidly will lead to acute locking, throwing the patient to the ground. In smaller lesions there are likely to be intermittent attacks with joint effusion and quadriceps wasting, as well as locking. The treatment is usually surgical. The introduction of the operating arthroscope has made the treatment much less traumatic.

Prepatellar bursitis

Housemaid's knee and clergyman's knee are common conditions in which there is inflammation of prepatellar or infrapatellar bursae. Usually the problem arises from chronic trauma with non-specific thickening of the bursa. From time to time the bursa becomes infected, perhaps from direct penetration of the bursa.

When this happens there will be a rapid increase in the swelling, with pain and generalised malaise. If there is no infection, the condition can be treated with steriod injection and by relieving the pressure on the knee. If infection is present, this is treated by aspiration and systemic antibiotics. In persistent cases, surgical removal may be necessary.

CHAPTER 9

PAIN IN THE FOOT AND ANKLE

Introduction

Pain in the foot must be one of the most miserable problems that a person can experience. Just as we depend on the hand to allow us to manipulate the environment, we depend on our feet to move us about that environment. Because the foot is frequently being stressed from walking, and the ankle is often being injured on rough ground, especially when running, there is excess trauma which will encourage the onset of osteoarthritis and act as a site for the onset of inflammatory arthritis. Frequently the foot is underestimated by the doctor and less attention is paid to the treatment of the problems that arise.

The History

This chapter will consider the ankle and foot together.

The important factors to discover in the history are as follows.

1   How long has the pain been present?
2   Is this the first episode of pain or have there been previous attacks?
3   Where is the pain?
4   What is the nature of the pain?
5   Is the pain worse at any particular time of day?
6   Is the pain worse on weight-bearing?
7   Does the pain limit walking?
8   Is there any swelling?
9   Is there any stiffness and, if so, when?
10   Was there an obvious precipitating cause?
11   Are there any other joints involved?
12   Is there any weakness?
13   Are there any paraesthesiae?
14   Are there any systemic symptoms?
15   Is there a significant past history?
16   Is there a significant family history?
17   What treatment has been tried and, if any, has it been effective?

In rheumatoid and other causes of erosive arthritis, metatarsophalangeal joint involvement will frequently lead to a history of a sensation like a pebble or broken glass in the shoe.

Reiter's syndrome frequently presents with pain in the feet and a careful enquiry about inflamed eyes, skin lesions, urethritis and diarrhoea is required.

The Examination

Once a satisfactory history has been obtained the ankle

and foot can be examined. It is important to remove socks or stockings. Both sides should be compared. No examination of the foot is complete without looking at the shoes for evidence of abnormal wear. The examination will be broken down into the various parts of the ankle and foot.

The nail

Table 9.1   Nail changes in the foot

Inspection	Palpation	Causes
Clubbing	Soft nail beds	Intrathoracic and intra-abdominal disease
Thickening	—	Onychogryphosis Psoriasis Fungal infection
Pitting	—	Psoriasis
Onycholysis	—	Psoriasis Chronic trauma Chronic infection
Nailfold infarcts	Tenderness	Vasculitis
Paronychia	Tenderness	Infection

Clubbing of the toes may be seen at the same time as in the fingers. However, it may be seen alone when there is an intra-abdominal cause. This may lead to hypertrophic pulmonary osteoarthropathy only in the legs.

Psoriatic nail changes will be seen in the toenails, and will have to be differentiated from fungal infections and onychogryphosis which can also distort the nail.

The skin

As inflammation resolves, particularly in gout,

there will be desquammation of the overlying skin.

Table 9.2   *Skin changes in the foot*

Inspection	Palpation	Cause
Erythema	Warm	Inflammatory arthritis Gout Infection
Oedema	Pitting, tender	Postural oedema Heart failure Low protein states, including nephrotic syndrome Rheumatoid arthritis Seronegative arthritis Gout Sepsis Trauma Lymphatic obstruction
Dusky	May be tender	Ischaemia Raynaud's phenomenon Algodystrophy
Ulceration	May be tender	Diabetes Vasculitis Venous insufficiency Trauma Infection
Gangrene	—	Peripheral vascular disease Diabetes Vasculitis

Oedema can arise from a number of causes in the foot. It is important to exclude heart failure and low protein states. It can also be a complication of acute arthritis but usually it is dependent, with no specific underlying cause.

Keratoderma blennorrhagica is the typical lesion of Reiter's syndrome. It looks very much like guttate psoriasis on the sole of the foot.

Bruising under either malleolus is due to rupture of the knee joint.

Raynaud's phenomenom can be seen in the feet and may be accompanied by cold damage, with gangrene. Gangrene may also be seen in diabetes, peripheral vascular disease and vasculitis.

The joints

Table 9.3   *Joint changes in the foot*

Inspection	Palpation	Causes
Erythema	Warm, tender	Rheumatoid arthritis Seronegative arthritis Gout Sepsis Trauma
Swelling	Tender	Osteoarthritis Rheumatoid arthritis Seronegative arthritis Gout (+ tophi) Oedema (Table 9.2)
Loss of function	Tender and crepitant	Osteoarthritis Rheumatoid arthritis Seronegative arthritis Gout Peripheral neuropathy Diabetes Trauma Sepsis Algodystrophy Morton's metatarsalgia Plantar fasciitis Achilles tendonitis
Deformity	—	Osteoarthritis Rheumatoid arthritis Seronegative arthritis Gout Trauma Nerve lesions

Ulcers around the ankle are seen in rheumatoid vasculitis. Unlike venous ulcers there is no eczema and pain is a major problem. Diabetic ulceration can occur on the sole of the foot and can lead to gangrene and osteomyelitis. Tophi on the toes can ulcerate, extruding monosodium urate.

Rheumatoid nodules are frequently seen around the Achilles tendon. Much less common is thickening in the sole due to Dupuytren's diathesis.

Callus forms as a response to abnormal, prolonged pressure. It is a good indication of disturbed anatomy but may just be due to ill-fitting footwear.

Tenderness of the metatarsophalangeal joints is a classical sign in rheumatoid arthritis and must always be sought if the diagnosis is suspected. The big toe should be ignored as it is so often the site of osteoarthritis. The other toes should all be firmly squeezed between the examiner's thumb and index finger. Tenderness in the heel may be due to an isolated plantar fasciitis or the enthesopathy of Reiter's syndrome. The Achilles tendon may also be inflamed in arthritis or following injury.

A complete foot-drop is obvious but minor weakness may be difficult to demonstrate. This is best done by getting the patient to stand up and then attempt to go on to his heels, which is impossible if there is weakness. Calf muscle weakness can be brought out by asking the patient to go on to tip-toe.

The plantar reflexes can be extremely difficult to analyse in patients with hallux valgus or previous forefoot surgery.

Details of the dermatomes which involve the lower leg and foot are given in Chapter 6.

Neurological system

Table 9.4　*Neurological signs in the foot*

Lesion	Physical signs	Cause
Tarsal tunnel syndrome	Sensory loss, medial three toes and sole	Rheumatoid arthritis Local trauma Idiopathic
Foot drop	Loss of dorsiflexion	Local trauma (neck of fibula) Peripheral neuropathy (see below) Nerve root compression (see below)
Nerve root compression	Foot drop, loss of ankle jerk, loss of sensation	Prolapsed intervertebral disc Spinal stenosis Herpes zoster Poliomyelitis Fracture Bony secondaries Sepsis
Mononeuritis multiplex	Any combination of nerve lesions	Diabetes Rheumatoid arthritis Polyarteritis nodosa Systemic lupus erythematosus Multiple sclerosis
Peripheral neuropathy	Loss of sensation in stocking distribution and motor weakness	Diabetes Rheumatoid arthritis Systemic lupus erythematosus Multiple sclerosis Subacute combined degeneration of the cord Toxins Guillain–Barré syndrome Non-metastatic malignant neuropathy Hereditary neuropathies

Investigating the Ankle and Foot

As most of the diseases seen in the foot and ankle form part of more generalised conditions the full investigation will not be discussed here (see Chapter 2), the emphasis being on the special tests that apply to this part of the body alone.

Blood tests

In patients with evidence of peripheral neuropathy or ulceration in the foot it is important to check the blood glucose (and to test the urine).

X-rays

Plain films of the foot are usually taken from above or obliquely to show the fore- and mid-foot in detail. If the ankle is being examined there will be a lateral film of the foot and ankle and an anteroposterior view through the ankle to show the mortice joint.

To count as erosions, the cortex of the bone must be breached. Erosions will appear in the feet long before anywhere else. Erosive change in the first metatarsophalangeal joint should be ignored if there are no erosions elsewhere as the joint is exposed constantly to trauma. Degenerative changes at this site can mimic erosions. The punched-out erosions of gout are fairly distinctive but the diagnosis should never have to depend on an X-ray alone.

The typical appearances are given in Table 9.5.

Table 9.5　X-ray appearances in the foot

Lesion	Site	Cause
Osteoporosis	Generalised	Disuse Infection Diabetes
	Patchy Periarticular	Sudeck's atrophy Inflammatory arthritis
Erosions	First MTP joints	Osteoarthritis Gout Rheumatoid arthritis
	2nd–5th MTP joints	Rheumatoid arthritis Seronegative arthritis
	Mid-foot Calcaneum	Rheumatoid arthritis Seronegative arthritis
Loss of joint space	First MTP joint	Osteoarthritis Gout Rheumatoid arthritis Seronegative arthritis
	2nd–5th MTP joints	Rheumatoid arthritis Seronegative arthritis Sepsis
	Mid-foot	Rheumatoid arthritis Seronegative arthritis Sepsis Bleeding disorders
	Hind-foot and Ankle	Rheumatoid arthritis Seronegative arthritis Osteoarthritis Bleeding disorders Sepsis
Deformity	Fore-foot	Osteoarthritis Rheumatoid arthritis Seronegative arthritis Gout Trauma Sepsis
	Mid-foot	Rheumatoid arthritis Trauma Sepsis Congenital abnormality Neurological lesions 　(including old 　poliomyelitis)

Table 9.5 (cont.) X-ray appearances in the foot

Lesion	Site	Cause
Deformity	Hind-foot and ankle	Rheumatoid arthritis Seronegative arthritis Trauma Sepsis Bleeding disorders
Cysts	Any	Osteoarthritis Gout Rheumatoid arthritis (pre-erosive)
Loss of bone	Any	Trauma Scleroderma Tumours Sepsis
Increased density	Any	Paget's disease of bone Tumour
Periosteal reaction	Any	Hypertrophic pulmonary osteoarthropathy Juvenile chronic arthritis Hyperparathyroidism Sepsis Bleeding disorders
Soft tissue calcification	Digits	Scleroderma
	Joints	Pyrophosphate deposition Gout
	Blood vessels	Diabetes Atherosclerosis

Loss of joint space due to infection will show involvement of the surrounding bone. That associated with osteoarthritis will show the presence of osteophytes. If the loss of joint space is due to inflammatory arthritis there will be periarticular osteoporosis.

It is common for the metatarsophalangeal joints to dislocate. The functional consequences of this can be better demonstrated by performing a tangential X-ray to show the position of the dropped metatarsal heads.

Electromyography (EMG)

EMG is very helpful in deciding the site of damage in foot-drop. It is possible to see if the anterior tibial nerve has been damaged as it winds around the neck of the fibula or whether it is involved in more widespread nerve damage. EMG can also be used to identify muscle abnormality in diseases such as dermatomyositis, although it is very rare for the foot to show signs of the disease.

Specific Conditions in the Foot and Ankle

Rheumatoid arthritis (RA)

Because RA tends to affect joints that are damaged or used frequently, the feet are often the site of major difficulty. The patients complain that they feel as if they are walking on broken glass or with a pebble in the shoe. Hallux valgus is common, with a large bunion forming. This makes the purchase of footwear difficult, compounding the difficulty with walking. There is likely to be dislocation of the metatarsophalangeal joints, with dropping of the metatarsal heads and flexion of the interphalangeal joints (Figure 9.1). This again makes footwear difficult to fit and may well lead to callus formation.

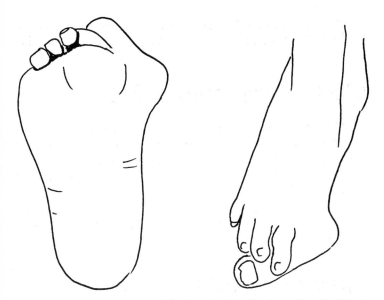

Figure 9.1 Distortion of the forefoot in rheumatoid arthritis

As the disease progresses joints in the tarsus and around the ankle will become involved. The result of this is a painful, swollen foot with instability of the ankle. It must be remembered that the ankle joint is a mortice between the distal ends of the tibia and fibula and the talus. This joint allows for dorsiflexion and plantar flexion. Inversion and eversion occur at the subtalar joint and it is often this joint which gives the most pain on walking, especially on uneven ground. It also means that treatment directed to the ankle joint alone (such as joint replacement) may do nothing for the most painful component of the foot. In late disease the valgus foot can be particularly distressing. The hind foot becomes everted and pressure starts to be taken on the medial border of the foot on walking.

Vasculitis may lead to painful, indolent ulcers

around the ankle and the stocking anaesthesia of peripheral neuropathy may be evident. Raynaud's syndrome and cold injury can occur. Hip disease may make cutting of the nails impossible.

When considering treatment there are a number of specific measures that can be applied to the foot and ankle other than the general therapy of the arthritis (see Chapter 12). The most important way of helping is to provide adequate footwear. A full surgical shoe or boot is required only in a small minority of patients. It is usually sufficient to provide a 'depth' shoe which will accommodate the dropped metatarsal heads and the flexed interphalangeal joints. It is also possible to supply a weight-distributing insole to fit in this type of shoe. Other helpful appliances are the metatarsal dome support for early disease and the ankle–foot orthosis to stabilise the painful subtalar joint.

The use of proper footwear will take pressure off painful areas in the foot. This is the correct way to deal with callus formation. Cutting the callus does nothing for the underlying problem and there is the risk of infection and ulceration.

The surgical reconstruction of the fore-foot is very successful. The correction of hallux valgus and the removal of metatarsal heads will usually provide a pain-free functional foot. Ankle surgery is less success-ful. Ankle replacement is beginning to be of value but the subtalar joint and the hind- and mid-foot can only be arthrodesed if they are to be made pain-free.

Ankylosing spondylitis (AS)

AS rarely causes a synovitis in the foot but plantar fasciitis and Achilles tendonitis are frequent. In the former condition there will be tenderness in the heel, with pain on weight-bearing. Achilles tendonitis gives pain on walking at the back of the ankle with tenderness and swelling at the same site.

Treatment of these two conditions is discussed below.

Reiter's syndrome

The foot usually bears the brunt of this disease. Achilles tendonitis, plantar fasciitis, and synovitis are all common, giving rise to considerable problems walking. X-rays will often show an exuberant plantar spur or erosive change at the insertion of the Achilles tendon into the calcaneum. The synovitis can affect any of the joints in the foot but there is a tendency for the metatarsophalangeal and interphalangeal joints to be worst affected. 'Sausage' toes are seen due to mild dactylitis.

Treatment is firstly to try to control the disease by the use of non-steroidal drugs. Next the Achilles tendon and plantar spur should be treated as mentioned below. Footwear may need to be modified and surgery advised for severe cases. Despite the optimistic prognosis given in many texts this disease is frequently recurrent and persistent.

Psoriasis

The feet can be involved in all three types of psoriatic arthritis. In the mild disease there is usually foot involvement, with 'sausage' toes and some metatarsalgia. In the mutilating form of the disease, pen-and-cup deformities may be seen in the toes and there is likely to be extensive destructive arthritis throughout the ankle and foot. In the spondylitic form, enthesopathy involving the Achilles tendon and plantar fascia will be seen.

Systemic lupus erythematosus (SLE)

SLE will cause trouble in the foot for a number of reasons. Firstly there will be arthritis, which is rarely erosive but can be very painful. Secondly there may be oedema associated with renal and cardiovascular disease and, lastly, there may be a peripheral neuritis with the whole range of motor and sensory signs.

Gout

The classical site for acute gout is the big toe – podogra. Most patients experience their first attack of gout in a big toe. They usually awake with an exquisitely painful, red and swollen toe. The toe is so tender that even the weight of the bedclothes cannot be tolerated and walking is impossible. The skin overlying the joint is dry. If untreated the attack will slowly subside over a week to 10 days. The ankle is also a common site for acute attacks.

The big toe is also a common site of chronic tophaceous gout. The metatarsal joint becomes eroded and may be disrupted. The skin over the tophus may ulcerate, extruding monosodium urate crystals.

The treatment of gout is discussed in Chapter 12.

Osteoarthritis (OA)

On X-ray, everyone over the age of 35 will have some evidence of degenerative change in the first metatarsophalangeal joint. Luckily, only a relatively small proportion of people get significant symptoms. Two problems are commonly seen. The first is hallux valgus in which there is a lateral deviation of the big toe, often with thickening of the soft tissues over the medial side of the joint – a bunion. This deformity is associated with the wearing of high-heeled shoes with narrow toes. The other problem is hallux rigidus in which there is loss of joint space with osteophyte formation. The toe is extremely painful to move, and walking (and especially running) are extremely painful. OA can occur at the ankle, again producing severe pain on walking.

Treatment of OA in the foot is to get the patient to lose weight, take simple analgesics and wear sensible shoes. For many this will be sufficient. However, a proportion will get persistent pain and surgery may be necessary. The first metatarsophalangeal joint can be excised or replaced with a silastic endoprosthesis. The ankle can be replaced or arthrodesed.

Arch abnormalities

Some people have completely flat feet all their lives while others have very high arches. When this is the case, symptoms in the feet are rarely due to the configuration of the foot. However, if the shape of the foot is changing rapidly then discomfort is likely. The longitudinal arch may collapse in inflammatory arthritis and this is commonplace with the transverse arch.

An arch support or custom-made insole will often relieve the symptoms.

The high-arch foot – pes cavus – can be due to a variety of neurological conditions in which there is muscle imbalance, such as Friedreich's ataxia. If there is increasing pes cavus it is important to exclude a neurological cause. The foot can usually be made more comfortable by the careful selection of footwear.

Tarsal tunnel syndrome

This is much less common than carpal tunnel syndrome. It presents as burning pain with paraesthesiae in the toes and sole of the foot. There is sensory loss in sole, but this is variable as one or more branches of the posterior tibial nerve can be compressed. The damage occurs in the tarsal tunnel which runs between the medial malleolus and the calcaneum.

It is treated either by steroid injection or surgical decompression.

Morton's metatarsalgia

In this condition patients present with pain and tenderness in the forefoot which makes walking unpleasant. There is no other evidence on history or examination of a more widespread arthritis. Careful examination of the foot will show that the tenderness is not in the joint but in the web space just by the metatarsophalangeal joint. It is due to the formation of a small neuroma on the digital nerve and responds to surgical excision.

Plantar fasciitis

This is one form of enthesopathy, where there is inflammation where the plantar fascia is inserted in the calcaneum. The story is one of pain on walking and of a discrete tender area in the heel. Some patients have evidence of a plantar spur on X-ray but so do many people who do not have symptoms. Similarly, quite a lot of symptomatic people have normal X-rays. The majority of patients have this as an isolated problem but it can complicate the seronegative arthropathies.

Treatment can be done in a number of ways. Frequently local steroid injection will abolish the pain. It is important to locate the area of maximum tenderness. It is inadvisable to inject the area through the sole, as this is most unpleasant for the patient, but to approach the heel from the side. It may need to be repeated several times. A heel pad is very helpful. It should be made out of a firm material, such as a high-density foam. The area of maximum tenderness is found and a hole cut out of the pad to take the weight off that area. In persistent cases surgical exploration of the heel may be necessary.

Achilles tendonitis

This can occur as an isolated lesion or part of an inflammatory arthritis, including seronegative arthritis. The back of the ankle will be swollen and painful, especially when running. Examination will show that the tendon is thickened and tender. It is important not to inject these as there is a very real risk of tendon rupture, which can be disastrous. Instead, the patient should be encouraged to rest, in plaster if necessary. Ultrasound may be beneficial.

Sever's disease

This is one of the forms of osteochondritis in which there is increased density in the posterior apophysis of the calcaneum. It causes pain in the heel predominantly in young children, and usually can be controlled by the use of an elevated heel on the shoe.

Diabetes

The foot can be compromised in a number of ways in diabetes. It can cause a peripheral neuropathy with painful paraesthesiae. Lack of sensation can lead to ulceration following minor penetrating injury which, in turn, can lead to infection and osteomyelitis. Vascular involvement may lead to gangrene. The foot is a common site for the diabetic form of neuropathic joint with considerable joint destruction. This means that all diabetics must be carefully coached in foot care. This includes regular visits to the chiropodist and daily inspection of the feet. This should include examining the sole of the foot with a mirror if the patient cannot inspect if directly.

March fracture

Clearly the foot is liable to considerable trauma, but this is not the place to review the majority of problems that can arise. However, march fracture can present as a chronic pain in the foot with no history of injury. There will be tenderness in the forefoot but careful palpation will show that the tenderness is not in the joint but in the shaft of the metatarsal. X-ray will show the fracture, usually in either the third or fourth metatarsal. Initially there will only be a hairline crack but abundant callus formation will later surround the crack. The pain will settle spontaneously but, while it is healing, it is best to stop the patient walking any more than is necessary.

CHAPTER 10

OTHER CONDITIONS

Introduction

This book is mainly centred around a regional approach to pain in the joints. This does lead to some conditions being overlooked and it is the function of this short chapter to fill the gap. The diseases mentioned below occur sufficiently frequently in rheumatological practice to be worthy of mention or to require expansion on the minor entries earlier in the book. For convenience they are mentioned in alphabetical order.

Acromegaly

This is due to an overproduction of growth hormone in adults. It is due to a pituitary adenoma. This produces an enlargement of the hands, feet and head. About half the patients will develop joint symptoms. Carpal tunnel syndrome is common. The features become coarse and the hands typically become huge. X-rays will show the exaggerated tufting of the terminal phalanges, together with bony outgrowths around the joint. A lateral view of the ankle can be used to measure the thickness of the heel pad. Skull X-ray should show enlargement of the pituitary fossa.

Treatment is by the surgical removal of the adenoma.

Amyloidosis

Amyloid is a term used to describe a group of proteins that form fibrils. These get laid down in extracellular tissues, sometimes in large waxy deposits, more often as infiltrates throughout various organs. The chemical composition of amyloid varies but in patients with multiple myeloma (see below) the protein is made of the terminal fragments of the light chains of immunoglobulins. Secondary amyloid is seen not only in myeloma but also in a range of chronic inflammatory conditions such as rheumatoid arthritis, juvenile chronic arthritis, tuberculosis, bronchiectasis, osteomyelitis and leprosy. It may also occur as primary disease with no predisposing condition.

Amyloid presents in a number of ways. It can give rise to a widespread polyarthritis, which closely resembles rheumatoid, including a high incidence of carpal tunnel syndrome. The involvement of internal organs leads to renal, hepatic and cardiac failure. Peripheral neuropathy is common. There is considerable overlap in the manifestations of the various types of amyloid but primary disease is more likely to present with large deposits in the tongue – macroglossia. Any patient with a chronic inflammatory condition who presents with proteinuria should be suspected of having amyloid. The diagnosis can usually be made on rectal biopsy.

Treatment is unsatisfactory. If there is an underlying cause this should be treated, but this rarely makes much difference. Immunosuppressive drugs have been tried (particularly melphalan) but the results are disappointing.

Behçet's Syndrome

This is an unusual condition in which there is arthritis, inflammatory eye disease, orogenital ulceration and central nervous system involvement, usually aseptic meningitis and stroke. The arthritis tends to be mild and non-deforming. The ulcers resemble large, indolent aphthous ulcers. The genital ulcers occur on the vulva or on the shaft of the penis. There are a range of eye complications, most notably anterior and posterior uveitis.

Treatment is a combination of symptomatic, with non-steroidal anti-inflammatory drugs and simple local treatment for the ulcers, together with systemic measures. Mild cases may be successfully controlled with colchicine while others will require immunosuppressives.

Erythema Nodosum

This manifests itself by the production of painful raised lumps on the legs, with the majority being below the knee. They tend to appear one or two at a time and fade away over the space of a week or 10 days leaving a characteristic bruised appearance to the skin. It is often accompanied by a mild synovitis, especially in the knees. It seems likely that the condition is an allergic or reactive one. Among the things that are known to precipitate it are sarcoidosis, tuberculosis, streptococcal infections and drugs of various sorts, including oral contraceptives. Most cases respond spontaneously and no treatment (other than to the underlying condition) is necessary. Occasionally it becomes persistent and troublesome and small doses of steroids are needed.

Familial Mediterranean Fever (FMF)

This condition, as its name suggests, is an hereditary, episodic condition seen in certain racial groups whose origin is in the Middle East, such as Jews, Armenians and Arabs. There are short-lived attacks of high fever, peritonitis, synovitis and pleurisy. Unless checked, amyloid will develop and death will ensue from renal failure. The arthritis tends to be an acute large-joint monarthritis. The attacks last up to a week. The diagnosis is made on the clinical picture and by finding the amyloid fibrils on electron microscopy of the urine.

The treatment of FMF is with colchicine, which will control the acute attacks and delay or stop the amyloid being precipitated.

Henoch–Schönlein Purpura

This is an allergic vasculitis in which there is purpura, fever, abdominal pain, arthralgia and renal disease.

The platelet count is normal. It is precipitated by streptococcal infection and drugs, including penicillin. The condition is seen mainly in adolescents and young adults. The purpuric rash occurs most profusely on the lower half of the body. Colicky abdominal pain is common. Joint pain is widespread but actual arthritis unusual. The renal disease, which is self-limiting as a rule, is a focal glomerulonephritis. Unless the renal disease becomes severe and persistent, the prognosis is good and general measures only are required. There is little evidence that steroids or immunosuppressives influence the condition much.

Multiple Myeloma

This is a fairly common malignant disease of plasma cells in which there are multiple deposits of a single clone of plasma cell which produces large quantities of monoclonal antibody, replaces bone marrow, erodes bone and leads to amyloidosis. Back pain is a common symptom. Bone pain elsewhere is also seen. The bone marrow replacement can lead to anaemia. The monoclonal antibody may interfere with coagulation or platelet function, leading to abnormal bleeding. The vast quantities of immunoglobulin produced can cause hyperviscosity syndrome. Protein turnover is such that urate levels may be increased and gout precipitated. Investigation includes the finding of the immunoglobulin in the blood (by electrophoresis) and in the urine (Bence–Jones's protein). The sedimentation rate is usually raised to high levels. X-ray will show punched-out lesions in bone, including the skull. Bone marrow aspiration will reveal large quantities of plasma cells. They may have normal morphology but abnormal forms are seen. The light chain immunoglobulins are the ideal size to form amyloid fibrils and this is a serious complication as renal failure is likely.

Treatment is two-pronged. Firstly the general physical condition of the patient is maintained. Adequate hydration is essential and such things as blood transfusion, analgesics and radiotherapy for bone pain are all valuable. Secondly chemotherapy, usually in the form of melphalan or cyclophosphamide, is of value and, if started early enough and managed skilfully, will improve the otherwise limited prognosis.

Myxoedema

This is mentioned as it can cause both muscle and joint symptoms, usually of aching pain, but a low-grade synovitis is seen, as is carpal tunnel syndrome. The musculoskeletal symptoms will subside if the hypothyroidism is adequately treated.

Psychogenic Rheumatism

Everybody feels pain every day. It is for most people a warning of present danger or past indiscretion and soon forgotten. However this everyday pain can be accentuated by physical or psychological illness, especially depression. Some people unconsciously use pain as a defence against an unacceptable lifestyle, while others use it to gain attention and sympathy. It is common for depressed people to have a minor musculoskeletal lesion which will act as a focus for pain. Many depressed people, particularly those not prone to showing emotion openly, will present with physical symptoms only, and it may be hard to explain to them the true nature of those symptoms. It must also be remembered that certain painful conditions, most notably polymyalgia rheumatica, will have depression as a clinical feature, while others, such as malignant bone pain, are depressing in themselves. However, if it is clear that psychological factors are playing a major role in the patient's illness, it is important not to ignore this. A clear explanation of the problem should be given to the patient and treatment offered, whether that be pharmacological or psychological.

Rheumatic Fever

Rheumatic fever is uncommon in Western industrial countries, probably due to a change in the nature of the streptococcus. It is still a frequent problem in some of the Third World countries. It must be recognised as it continues to be seen occasionally. As the disease has evolved the age group at risk from the first attack has risen, so that it is more likely now to be seen in late adolescence. Second attacks can occur in the 20s. The history is of a severe flitting polyarthritis, fever, malaise and a rash – erythema marginatum. The arthritis moves from joint to joint but the migratory nature of it will disappear if the patient is given aspirin or a non-steroidal agent. The involved joint is swollen and extremely tender. Patients may complain of breathlessness, and heart valve lesions must be actively sought. This will mean repeated auscultation. Many patients will give a history of a previous sore throat and a group A beta-haemolytic streptococcus may be grown on throat swab. Most patients will have a raised

ASO titre as evidence of a recent streptococcal infection.

Treatment depends on the presence or absence of carditis. If absent then aspirin and joint aspiration are sufficient but if carditis does develop, bed-rest is sensible. Steroids are of doubtful help. It may be necessary to consider emergency valve replacement if severe valve damage occurs. In either case penicillin should be given to eliminate any residual streptococci. If carditis does occur it is important to remember that the patient should take prophylactic antibiotics to prevent further attacks and to cover any manipulations that are likely to produce a bacteraemia, such as dental extraction or sigmoidoscopy.

Tietze's Syndrome

This is a condition in which there is pain and tenderness in one or more costosternal junctions. It is important to recognise as patients become convinced that they have heart or lung disease. Investigations are normal, and patients can be strongly reassured about the benign nature of the condition. It is self-limiting but, if it is a persistent problem, the tender area can be injected with local steroids.

CHAPTER 11

ARTHRITIS IN CHILDREN

Introduction

The purpose of this short chapter is to draw attention
to the spectrum of rheumatological conditions that can
be seen in children. It is not a comprehensive text and
readers interested in this topic are strongly advised to
consult one or more of the larger works mentioned in
the Further Reading list. Arthritis is not particularly
common, there probably being 15 000 to 20 000 cases
in the UK at any one time and up to 200 000 cases in
the USA. Because it is uncommon it is not always
diagnosed or treated properly. There has also been
considerable confusion in the past over the nomencla-
ture, a confusion which still prevails in North America.
For a long time all arthritis in childhood was described
as Still's disease and then as juvenile rheumatoid
arthritis. The first term is obscure and open to
misinterpretation as Still described what is now recognised as the systemic form of juvenile chronic arthritis
(JCA). The second term is wrong because JCA is not
rheumatoid arthritis occurring in children, there being

major clinical and investigational differences. What is more, there is true rheumatoid arthritis occurring in children.

Juvenile Chronic Arthritis (JCA)

JCA is defined as arthritis occurring under the age of 16 and persisting for at least 3 months. The age cut-off is arbitrary. The time requirement is put in to avoid diagnosing JCA in patients with post-viral and other self-limiting arthropathies. Three distinct subsets are recognised:

1 systemic
2 polyarticular
3 pauciarticular.

Systemic Disease

This approximates most closely to what Still described. It can come at any time from the first months of life to about 8 years old. At the time of onset the child is ill with fever; general malaise; a characteristic red, slightly raised evanescent rash, mainly visible on the trunk; and lymphadenopathy. The arthritis may be quite inconspicuous initially, leading to considerable diagnostic confusion. However, as time progresses, it becomes more obviously a polyarthritis. At presentation about half the patients have splenomegaly, while hepatomegaly and pericardial effusion are seen less frequently. This is a serious illness which still carries a small risk of a fatal outcome. Many of these patients will be of small stature, independent of steroid treatment. Like the majority of JCA sufferers, the patients in this subgroup have a good prognosis in the sense that the disease will go into remission but the stigmata of the joint disease will be carried into adult life.

Polyarticular Disease

This also occurs in the younger age group. Presentation is with a widespread polyarthritis, particularly involving the hands, feet, knees and cervical spine. There will be pain, stiffness, swelling and deformity. Often there are growth inequalities of bone, including those of the fingers and jaw, leading to further deformity. The grossly underdeveloped jaw is a typical finding. As with the systemic disease, the overall prognosis is good but patients will carry any deformities through into later life.

Pauciarticular Disease

This is defined as four or less joints involved within the first 3 months of presentation. Usually it is the large joints, especially the knee, that are involved. There are three subgroups within the pauciarticular group, which all carry different outcomes, and it is important to recognise these. Over half have the presence of antinuclear antigen in the blood and up to a half of these will develop chronic anterior uveitis. This eye complication is so insidious that unless positive steps are taken to identify it the first complaint will be of loss of vision (see below). If eye disease does not occur the prognosis is very good. The other large subgroup is the antinuclear antigen-negative group. Chronic uveitis very rarely occurs with these children and overall the prognosis is good with virtually no likelihood of long-term joint problems. The last subgroup does have a poor prognosis. Although presenting as a pauciarticular condition, new joints became involved one or two at a time for many years. The result is widespread destructive arthritis that continues to be active well into adult life. Although they are numerically a very small group they are among the most disabled of all JCA sufferers.

Investigating Juvenile Chronic Arthritis

Care should be taken when investigating children. They do not like needles, and over-exposure to X-rays is potentially more harmful than in adults. No test should be done unless there is a positive diagnostic or management reason for doing it. In this section the emphasis is on those tests that are relevant to JCA. It is important to be aware of the differences in the normal values of such things as alkaline phosphatase, which vary at different ages and which can cause confusion. If in doubt ask the laboratory for advice.

Haematology

(a) *Haemoglobin*. There is likely to be an anaemia of chronic inflammation that is normochromic and normocytic.

(b) *White cells*. Children frequently have high white cell counts but JCA can push this up quite significantly, on occasions being in excess of 50 000 per mm^3.

(c) *Platelets*. These, too, may be elevated in active JCA.

(d) *Sedimentation rate*. The ESR will usually be elevated in JCA, as will the other non-specific measures such as plasma viscosity and c-reactive protein.

Immunology

(a) *Rheumatoid factor*. The rheumatoid factor is, almost by definition, negative in JCA. If it is positive then the diagnosis is juvenile rheumatoid arthritis (see below).

(b) *Antinuclear antigen*. This is an important test to do in pauciarticular JCA. If it is positive, considerable care must be taken to ensure that chronic anterior uveitis does not develop.

Urine tests

Patients with JCA run the risk of developing amyloidosis and thus regular tests for protein are needed.

X-rays

The typical X-ray lesion in early JCA is dactylitis with periosteal reaction rather than erosion. Joint inflammation hastens maturation of the affected bone and this leads to premature fusion of the epiphyses, which is the cause of growth inequality. As the disease progresses, affected joints will tend to fuse. One of the hallmarks of old disease is an entirely fused carpus.

Synovial fluid

This will show an inflammatory pattern similar to that seen in rheumatoid arthritis.

Slit lamp examination of the eye

All children with JCA should have their eyes examined by slit lamp at regular intervals. How long those intervals should be depends on the type of JCA. In the ANA-positive disease this should be done every 6 months. In systemic onset, particularly if there are continuing systemic symptoms, it should be done annually, as it should with ANA-negative pauciarticular patients. The polyarticular patients can probably be screened every 2 years or so.

Adult Still's Disease

A group of patients have been described who have many of the features of systemic JCA but who are adult, often in the 20s and 30s. Most are women. They have the typical rash, arthritis, and fever. Pleurisy, pericarditis and splenomegaly are all seen. It usually resolves spontaneously after several months but can relapse. The patients are quite ill with the condition but do respond to high-dose aspirin or non-steroidal agents.

Juvenile Rheumatoid Arthritis

This is a distinct clinical entity. It is rheumatoid arthritis starting before the age of 16. The majority of cases occur in the early teens but rarely it may be seen before the age of 10. The patients are rheumatoid factor positive. The prognosis is poor, particularly when compared to most cases of JCA. Many of these patients will have active, destructive rheumatoid arthritis for many years. They will require aggressive second-line therapy (see Chapter 12) from early on in their illness.

Juvenile Ankylosing Spondylitis

Just as rheumatoid arthritis may present in children, so may ankylosing spondylitis. However, backache is a very rare complaint in children and the majority of juvenile spondylitics present with peripheral arthritis, which, as it is seronegative, will be called JCA. X-rays of the sacroiliac joints will not help as those joints all look as if they are inflamed when young. A family history might help but the presence or absence of HLA B-27 is only of use in population studies. It means that if a boy presents with JCA after the age of 10 or 11 then the possibility of ankylosing spondylitis should be borne in mind and the patient followed with care into early adult life. If this is done, and the appropriate drug and physical treatment offered, the prognosis is quite good.

Juvenile Psoriatic Arthritis

This is another adult condition that occurs in children and tends to have a poor prognosis as the subset is frequently of the mutilating variety. The arthritis usually comes on after the psoriasis, which is likely to be extensive. These patients need to be followed most carefully and may need to be treated with drugs such as methotrexate.

Back Pain in Children

Young children do not get benign back pain. If a child under the age of 10 complains of back pain it is important to exclude infection or malignancy. Even in the teenager the complaint is uncommon, with Scheuermann's osteochondritis (see Chapter 6) being the only common example. Some children may complain of back pain if other members of the family are suffering from it, or may use it as an attention-seeking device.

Other Causes of Rheumatic Disease in Childhood

Table 11.1 gives details of the more important prob-

lems encountered in children. The list is not exhaustive
but gives an idea of the range of problems encountered.

Table 11.1   Causes of joint disorder in children

Rheumatic disorders	*Neoplastic disease*
Juvenile chronic arthritis	Leukaemia
Rheumatoid arthritis	Lymphoma
Rheumatic fever	Neuroblastoma
Systemic lupus erythematosus	
Anaphylactoid purpura	*Metabolic*
Systemic vasculitis	Lesch–Nyhan syndrome
Erythema nodosum	Hypothyroidism
Dermatomyositis	Hypoparathyroidism
Scleroderma	
Mixed connective tissue disease	*Inherited disease*
Ankylosing spondylitis	Sickle cell disease
Ulcerative colitis	Marfan's syndrome
Crohn's disease	Familial Mediterranean fever
Psoriasis	Epiphyseal dysplasia
Sarcoidosis	Ehlers–Danlos syndrome
Reiter's syndrome	Homocystinuria
Stevens–Johnson syndrome	Haemophilia
Behçet's syndrome	Immune deficiency syndromes
Polyarteritis nodosa	
	Miscellaneous
Infection	Transient synovitis
Septic arthritis	Palindromic rheumatism
Gonococcus	Trauma
Tuberculosis	Villonodular synovitis
Lyme disease	Osteochondritis
Rubella	Osteoid osteoma
Parvovirus	Tietze's syndrome
Hepatitis	Periodic fever
Mumps	Histiocytosis
Osteomyelitis	Juvenile osteoporosis
	Algodystrophy
	Psychogenic rheumatism

CHAPTER 12

TREATMENT OF THE RHEUMATIC DISEASES

Introduction

The object of this chapter is to outline the general approach to treating the rheumatic diseases. It is divided into three sections:

1. Drug therapy
   analgesics
   non-steroidal anti-inflammatory drugs
   specific drug therapy.
2. Physical treatment
   physiotherapy
   occupational therapy
   social intervention.
3. Surgery.

Because of the size and objectives of this book, most of the topics will be covered in broad outline rather than fine detail. There is a bias to discussion of the drug therapy but this does not mean that the physical side is any less important and clearly, in patients with late, disabling arthritis, the physical and social considerations will be the most important. It should also be stressed that the best results are obtained from a team approach that gives full professional recognition to the therapists, nurses, social workers, etc. who have a major role in management.

Drug therapy

Simple analgesics

Pain is the overwhelming complaint of patients with rheumatic conditions. Specific therapies may be available but often the careful use of a simple analgesic will make life bearable and help with the simple tasks of living, including sleeping. Table 12.1 lists the simple analgesics in common use in rheumatology.

Paracetamol remains the most useful of the simple analgesics. Its action is entirely peripheral, it does not adversely affect the gastric mucosa and it is a good occasional analgesic. Its drawbacks are that it is relatively weak and is highly dangerous in overdose.

Combination analgesics clearly have a place, if for no other reason than that they are extremely popular with patients. Dextropropoxyphene is centrally active and this may account for its success. These combinations are not good occasional analgesics and should be used in regular dosage for a better effect than just giving paracetamol alone.

Aspirin is included in this list for completeness, although clearly it has marked anti-inflammatory action. However many patients still use it as a additional analgesic in small doses.

There are some new so-called analgesics on the market. They are in reality non-steroidal agents that

Table 12.1   Simple analgesics

Official name	Dosage
*Preparations of aspirin**	
Aspirin	600–1200 mg. q.d.s.
Dispersible (soluble) aspirin	600–1200 mg. q.d.s.
Effervescent aspirin	600–1200 mg. q.d.s.
Enteric-coated aspirin	600–1200 mg q.d.s.
Slow-release aspirin	500–1000 mg q.d.s.
	648–1296 mg q.d.s.
Aloxiprin	600 mg per 6.5 kg body weight
Choline magnesium trisalicylate	1000–1500 mg b.d.
Salicyl-salicylic acid	500–1000 mg. q.d.s.
Aspirin/paracetamol mixtures	1–3 tabs q.d.s.
Benorylate	5–10 ml b.d.
Diflunisal	250–500 mg. b.d.
Other simple analgesics	
Benorylate	5–10 ml b.d.
Dextropropoxyphene	65 mg t.d.s–q.d.s.
Dextropropoxyphene mixtures	1–2 tabs q.d.s.
Dihydrocodeine	30 mg q.d.s.
Dihydrocodeine mixtures	1 tab 4-hourly
Suprofen	200 mg t.d.s or q.d.s.
Meptazinol	200 mg 3–6-hourly
Nefopam	60–90 mg t.d.s.

*Aspirin is also found in a wide range of analgesic mixtures, cold remedies and other 'over-the-counter' medicines.

are being promoted for pain alone. They have the same problems as other non-steroidals (see over).

The strong analgesics such as morphine have no place in the treatment of most chronic conditions but this needs to be reconsidered in patients with unremitting pain from, say, mutilating psoriatic arthritis that has not responded to any other form of treatment, drug, surgical or physical.

Non-steroidal anti-inflammatory drugs (NSAIDs)

Until recently NSAIDs were the fastest-growing group of pharmacological agents entering the market. They represent the mainstay of treatment in most rheumatic conditions. Although they can all be demonstrated to be anti-inflammatory in animals, they seem to work in man mainly by acting as potent and convenient analgesics. There is no good evidence that they modify the outcome of progressive diseases such as rheumatoid arthritis. Table 12.2 lists NSAIDs in common use at this time.

Aspirin was the original NSAID. It is a peripherally acting analgesic with marked anti-inflammatory effects in that it can reduce fever. It does not affect the outcome of inflammatory arthritis. Aspirin has several drawbacks. Large doses are needed to obtain the best effect and, as it has a short half-life, it needs to be taken regularly. It is very irritating on the stomach, producing contact bleeding. It does not have a systemic effect on the gastric mucosa like the majority of NSAIDs, however (see below). In overdose it is very dangerous and in doses required to relieve severe pain, it is likely to produce tinnitus and deafness, especially in the elderly. Although it is uricosuric in high dose, it causes uric acid retention in low dose and should not, therefore, be used in gout as it usually makes it worse. Because of the irritant effects on the stomach a number of alternative preparations are available which are better tolerated.

Despite the high incidence of side-effects, indomethacin is probably the best of the non-aspirin NSAIDs. It consistently gives good pain relief and is helpful with morning stiffness. The slow-release form has super-

Table 12.2 *Non-steroidal agents*

Official name	Dosage*	Advantages	Disadvantages
Indomethacin	75–150 mg daily Slow-release and suppositories available	Highly effective; especially good for morning stiffness	High incidence of side-effects, such as indigestion, gastrointestinal bleeding and headache
Phenylbutazone	100–300 mg daily	Good analgesic and anti-inflammatory	Dangerous in the elderly – pancytopenia, oedema
Naproxen	500–1000 mg daily	Little indigestion	Gastric bleeding
Ibuprofen	400 mg t.d.s. – 800 mg q.d.s.	Low incidence of side-effects	Weak agent, and side-effects increase if effective dose is given
Piroxicam	20 mg nocte with the addition of 10–20 mg mane	Convenient once- or twice-daily dosage, good for morning stiffness	Gastric ulceration often silent
Ketoprofen	100 mg–200 mg daily	Slow-release form available	Frequent indigestion
Fenbufen	600 mg nocte plus 300 mg mane if required	Low incidence of indigestion; well tolerated in the elderly	Skin rash
Sulidac	200 mg b.d.	Useful in renal impairment	Relatively weak agent
Fenoprofen	300–600 mg t.d.s. – q.d.s.		Absorption inhibited by food
Flurbiprofen	50–100 mg t.d.s.		Indigestion
Mefanamic acid	500 mg t.d.s. Good analgesic, non-constipating	Strongly anti-inflammatory	Diarrhoea
Azapropazone	1200 mg in divided doses	Uricosuric, may be drug of first choice in acute gout	Gastric ulceration
Tiaprofenic acid	600 mg daily in divided doses	Short half-life, therefore may be less damaging to the gut	—
Diclofenac	25–50 mg t.d.s.	Good enteric coating	Headache
Tolmetin	400 mg t.d.s.	Well tolerated	Displaced by aspirin

*Dosages are for guidance only. They may need to be increased in active inflammatory disease (especially gout), and will be lower in the elderly and in patients with general poor health.

seded the suppository which many patients find difficult to insert and retain. The major problem with the
drug is indigestion and gastric ulceration. The indigestion is probably related to direct gastric irritation but
the ulceration is a systemic effect (as it is with all
NSAIDs except aspirin) due to the inhibition of
protective prostaglandins. It therefore does not matter
if the drug is given orally, in an enteric coating or
rectally. Indigestion and ulceration do not co-relate.
The other important group of side-effects is in the
central nervous system, including headaches and dizzi-
ness. This gets worse the older the patient. It may
make driving and operating machinery dangerous.

If indomethacin is not tolerated there is a wide range
of alternatives available. The doctor should become
familiar with three or four of them. Often it is useful to
ask the patient to spend a fortnight on each of a 'panel'
of NSAIDs, choosing at the end the one that suits him
or her best. Usually it is a balance between effectiveness and side-effects that helps the patient decide
which one is best. None of these drugs can be regarded
as a panacea and the patients soon learn that they are
likely to be left with a residue of pain. It is important to
give a dose last thing at night to help with morning
stiffness if it is present. Apart from gastrointestinal
and central nervous system side-effects, the most
consistent problem with NSAIDs is skin rash, often
photosensitive.

Phenylbutazone is now only available from hospitals
for the treatment of ankylosing spondylitis.

Specific drug treatments

Gold

This is used in the treatment of rheumatoid arthritis

and psoriatic arthritis. It is probably best in early disease and can be successfully used in seronegative rheumatoid arthritis, which penicillamine cannot. It is a dangerous drug if not used carefully. Although an oral form of the drug has recently been marketed it is not as effective as the injections. Normally two or three test doses of the drug are given to ensure that there is no immediate allergic reaction. Then 50 mg is given weekly by intramuscular injection. This is continued until a response is seen, usually between 400 and 600 mg. At this point the dosage is reduced to 50 mg fortnightly and a further reduction at about 1 g to 50 mg monthly. If remission or control is obtained the treatment should be continued indefinitely as if it is stopped relapse is almost certain and second and subsequent 'courses' are never as effective. Should the patient start to relapse when the dose is reduced to fortnightly or monthly the frequency of the injections should be increased.

Monitoring is essential. There are three major side-effects.

1. *Skin rash*. This usually starts as an irritation, and exfoliative dermatitis can appear. This can be dramatic and even life-threatening. Thus, before every injection, an enquiry about the skin should be made and, if significant itch or rash is present, the injection should be withheld. However, if care is taken, about half the patients who complain of rash will be able to go back on the gold when the skin problem subsides.

2. *Bone marrow suppression*. This is the most dangerous side-effect with gold. Either a thrombocytopenia or neutropenia will be seen. Rarely will total marrow aplasia be seen. A careful check must be kept on the blood. The most convenient way of doing this is to take

a blood sample at the time the gold injection is given. The doctor should also be aware of the possibility of abnormal bruising, bleeding, and oral ulceration and sore throat. He should withhold the injection until the blood result is available if there is a clinical suspicion of bone marrow suppression. Sudden drops in the white cell and platelet count can occur, and a normal blood test from only the previous day may not show the true picture. However, it is safe to continue gold therapy if the white cell count remains above 3500 per cubic millimetre, with a neutrophil count in excess of 2500. The platelet count should be above 125 000 per cubic millimetre. It must be remembered that an elevated platelet count is a sign of active rheumatoid arthritis and a falling count evidence of improvement. Concern is only necessary when the count drops below 150 000.

3. *Nephrotic syndrome.* Gold can form complexes with immunoglobulins which are laid down in the basement membrane of the glomerulus, leading to a considerable protein leak. As a rule this will not affect renal function as such but frank nephrotic syndrome is likely. Before each injection the urine should be checked for protein. If there is more than trace or 1+ on dip-testing the injection should be withheld until a 24 hour urine test has been done. If the total protein is less than 750 mg then it is safe to proceed. If the loss is greater than 750 mg then a creatinine clearance test should be done and if the renal function is good and there is not frank nephrotic syndrome then it is safe to proceed. It has become clear that gold therapy can be continued if there is a good response and a benign protein leak.

As many patients on gold therapy are receiving joint care between hospital and general practice, it is sensible to use a cooperation card on which all the details of treatment and test results can be recorded.

D-penicillamine

This drug is used in the treatment of rheumatoid arthritis. It is probably best for seropositive disease, especially late disease. It is given orally and, like gold, needs to be given with great care. The best results are obtained by starting with a low dose, slowly building up. This will ensure that side-effects and dosage can be kept to a minimum. The starting dose is 125 mg. After 6 weeks this can be increased to 250 mg daily. At least one-third of patients will be improving significantly and no further increase will be needed. However, another increment may be needed. It is rare for the dose to be pushed up higher than 500 mg.

The serious side-effects are similar to those of gold but there are some that are not seen with any other agent commonly used. Bone marrow suppression is the most serious problem and blood tests at least every 4 weeks should be undertaken. Proteinuria is more common than with gold, but tends to be less serious and, as long as renal function remains within normal limits, it is safe to continue. Rash is less common but a pemphigus-like lesion is produced which leads to the withdrawal of the drug. A variety of more bizarre side-effects occur such as myasthenia gravis and drug-induced systemic lupus erythematosus. Patients on penicillamine should be encouraged to report any significant clinical event to the doctor in case it represents toxicity.

Anti-malarials

Chloroquine and hydroxychloroquine have been used successfully for many years to treat rheumatoid arthritis and systemic lupus erythematosus. Hydroxychloroquine is probably safer and should be regarded as the drug of first choice in this group. They are the safest of the second-line agents and the warnings about ocular toxicity much exaggerated. The retinopathy is not seen if the annual dose is kept below 100 g of hydroxychloroquine, which can be achieved by giving 200 mg twice a day for the first 3 months of treatment and then 200 mg daily. Using this regimen eye checks are unnecessary. It is also unnecessary to restrict the course of treatment to 1 or 2 years. The anti-malarials are the weakest of the second-line agents and have a place in controlling disease in patients with few symptoms but evidence of disease progression, or where regular blood and urine tests may be difficult.

Azathioprine

This is the safest of the immunosuppressive drugs. It is used as a second-line agent, with equivalent effectiveness to gold, and as a steroid-sparing agent. Steroids are quite undesirable in most rheumatic conditions; hence azathioprine is frequently valuable. The dosage is usually 2.5 mg per kg body weight. This is quite close to the toxic level and careful monitoring of the white cell and platelet counts is essential. However, if bone marrow suppression does occur, the drug usually only needs to be stopped for about a week and then restarted at a slightly lower dose. Macrocytosis is often seen but is benign. Nausea is frequent at the start of treatment but will wear off if the patient is encouraged to continue.

Other immunosuppressives

A variety of other agents are used in the rheumatic diseases, and are listed in Table 12.3.

Table 12.3   *Immunosuppressive drugs*

Drug	Dosage	Uses
Azathioprine	2.5 mg/kg daily	Rheumatoid arthritis Systemic lupus erythematosus Reiter's syndrome Polymyalgia rheumatica Steroid-sparing generally
Cyclophosphamide	1.5 mg/kg daily	Systemic lupus erythematosus Rheumatoid arthritis
Chlorambucil	0.5–1.5 mg/kg daily	Rheumatoid arthritis
Methotrexate	5–20 mg weekly	Psoriatic arthritis Dermatomyositis Rheumatoid arthritis

As with azathioprine, care must be taken with dosage and monitoring. In the rheumatic diseases there is little evidence that these drugs precipitate malignant disease, unlike in transplant patients. It is not uncommon for herpes zoster to be precipitated by any of the group. Methotrexate should be avoided in patients with pre-existing liver damage, especially if alcohol-induced. Cyclophosphamide can irritate the bladder and cause haemorrhagic cystitis and, rarely, bladder cancer. It can also cause sterility in men.

Sulphasalazine

This drug has recently attracted a renewed interest in the treatment of rheumatoid arthritis. It appears to be an effective second-line agent which is reasonably well tolerated, although gastrointestinal upset, hepatitis, oligospermia and allergic skin reactions can be troublesome. The urine may become orange-coloured.

Dosage is usually 500 mg daily initially, building up in 500 mg increments to 2 g a day. It is best to use the enteric-coated tablet.

Steroids

Although initially producing miraculous results in most rheumatic conditions, steroids frequently produce totally unacceptable side-effects. These include Cushingoid features, thinning of the skin, precipitation of diabetes, cataract, heart failure, peripheral vascular disease, osteoporosis, and peptic ulceration. With the last-mentioned this may be more a prevention of healing rather than a causation. The major problem, which can be life-threatening, is adrenal suppression. Steroids can also totally mask the signs and symptoms of peritonitis and similar catastrophes. There are times when steroids are clearly indicated. These include temporal arteritis, polymyalgia rheumatica, severe systemic lupus erythematosus, polyarteritis nodosa, many cases of polymyositis and dermatomyositis, and some complications of the rheumatic diseases, such as aggressive anterior uveitis in ankylosing spondylitis or fibrosing alveolitis in rheumatoid arthritis.

Prednisolone is probably the only drug worth considering for systemic use. It is easy to vary the dosage and does not cause a significant amount of muscle-wasting or fluid retention in dosages normally used in most rheumatological conditions. Every effort must be made to keep the dose to the lowest possible to control the disease process being treated. Less adrenal suppression may be produced if the drug is given as a single daily dose in the morning. If it is essential to treat children with steroids (because of severe systemic illness) then alternate-day therapy will help to prevent stunting of growth. If adults are on steroids azathioprine should be considered as a steroid-sparing agent, especially if unacceptable side-effects occur.

There is a place for using large doses of intravenous steroids in very active disease, such as rheumatoid arthritis, while initiating second-line therapy. It is usually given as a slow infusion of 1 g of methylprednisolone, perhaps repeated once or twice over the course of a week.

Allopurinol

This is the treatment of choice of recurrent gout. By blocking the formation of urate from xanthine, which is easily excreted by the kidney, the total body load of urate is reduced and tophi will be dissolved. It is a safe and easy drug to use, the only side-effect of significance being skin rash in a tiny minority of patients. However, it is best to start therapy only when there are clear-cut repeated attacks, tophi formation or renal impairment. One attack every 3 or 4 years that is easily controlled with a non-steroidal agent does not require the use of allopurinol. It is important to start the therapy when there is an absence of an acute attack. This is because the drug mobilises urate stores which can prolong and worsen an attack. For the same reason when treatment is initiated the patient must be given adequate cover with colchicine or a non-steroidal agent, such as azapropazone. It is usual to start with 100 mg daily of allopurinol, building up to 300 mg over the next 2 or 3 weeks. This will be sufficient for most patients but if the serum urate is still raised then the dose can be increased. After 8 weeks the covering colchicine or non-steroidal can be stopped. It must be impressed on the patient that he will need to continue on the allopurinol indefinitely, even if there has been no attack for some years.

Other treatments for gout

Colchicine can still be used for the acute attack of gout and to cover the initiation of allopurinol therapy. In acute gout 1 mg is given initially followed by 0.5 mg every 2–3 hours until either the attack subsides or diarrhoea or vomiting occurs. It is the gastrointestinal side-effects that really limit the usefulness of this drug. In the initiating of allopurinol therapy 0.5 mg twice a day is sufficient and is usually tolerated.

Uricosurics are not frequently used now, but may be required in patients with intolerance to allopurinol or in whom allopurinol is insufficient to control the disease. Probenicid is the most commonly used but sulphinpyrazone has its supporters. It is essential for the patient to maintain an adequate fluid intake and it is advisable to alkalinise the urine. Salicylates must be avoided.

Azapropazone is a non-steroidal anti-inflammatory drug that has uricosuric properties and is therefore probably the NSAID of first choice in the treatment of acute and chronic gout.

Calcitonin

Paget's disease of bone can be painful and in the skull can press on cranial nerves. Pain will not always be kept under control with simple analgesics, while the bone expansion may require specific treatment. Although there is a relative lack of good controlled data on effectiveness, calcitonin is the most popular drug for this purpose. It was originally derived from either pigs or salmon. Salmon calcitonin is now synthetic. It is given by injection. The treatment is very expensive and should not be pursued if a good result is not obtained quickly. A typical regimen would be 50 or 100 international units of the salmon preparation three times a week, given intramuscularly. It may cause flushing and nausea. Local irritation at the injection site is common and severe allergic reactions, including anaphylactic shock, may be seen in patients with a previous history of allergy. In this case a scratch test should be performed prior to the course. Normally courses should last up to 6 months, but can be repeated if there is relapse later. Salmon calcitonin has the major advantage that it is much less likely to cause the production of antibodies which can render the treatment ineffectual.

Disodium etidronate

This drug is a diphosphonate, a group of detergent-like drugs that get absorbed onto hydroxyapatite crystals, thus slowing down the rate of turnover of bone. It is used in the treatment of Paget's disease of bone. The normal dosage is 5 mg per kg body weight for 6 months, or 10 mg per kg for 3 months. Using the drug for longer periods of time will lead to significant weakening of bone with a high risk of pathological fracture. Because of its chemical properties it must not be given with food, especially calcium- or mineral-containing products. There must be a minimum period of 3 months between courses.

Injection therapy

Intra-articular and intra-lesional steroid injection is probably the most useful form of treatment available to the rheumatologist. Effusions can be drained and inflammation suppressed with the rapid resolution of pain and loss of function. Its use in the rheumatoid knee has seen the virtual disappearance of the fixed flexion deformity. The misery of tennis elbow and capsulitis of the shoulder can be abolished. Space precludes a full description of the whole range of possible injections. A description of knee injection is given in Chapter 8. The diagrams (Figures 12.1 to 12.6) show some of the most useful. Deep injections (e.g. knee and shoulder) can be made using triamcinolone hexacetonide but it is inadvisable to use this for superficial lesions (e.g. tennis elbow) because of the considerable amount of tissue atrophy associated with triamcinolone. With the exception of carpal tunnel syndrome it is normal to mix local anaesthetic with the steroid to (a) produce an immediate pain-relieving effect and (b) help spread the steroid throughout the joint. It is not necessary to take the patient to the operating theatre to perform intra-articular injections,

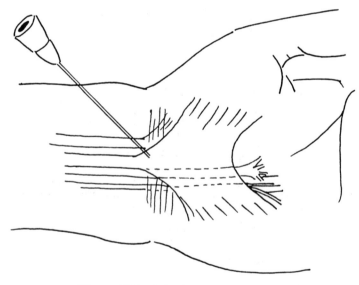

Figure 12.1   Injecting the carpal tunnel

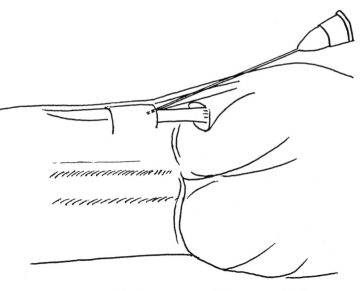

Figure 12.2   Injecting de Quervains's tenovaginitis

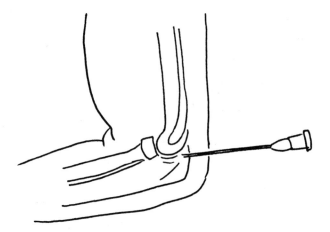

Figure 12.3   Injecting lateral epicondylitis

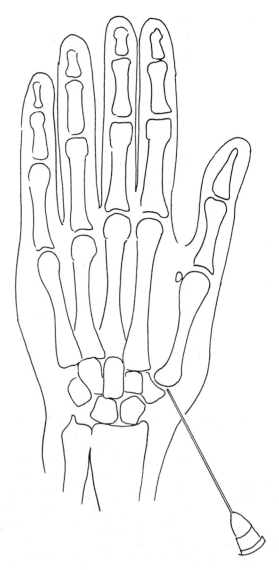

Figure 12.4   Injecting first C.M.C. osteo-arthritis

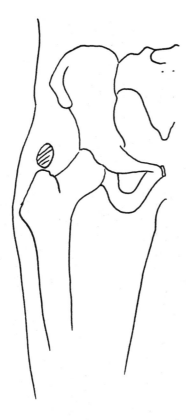

Figure 12.5   Site of trochanteric bursitis

a no-touch technique being adequate to prevent sepsis. As a rule of thumb, no joint or lesion should be injected more than three times in a 12-month period. Great care should be taken not to inject into a tendon, as rupture is likely. The Achilles tendon is particularly vulnerable. Patients should be warned that the injection may take up to 72 hours to work, and that the pain may get worse before it gets better.

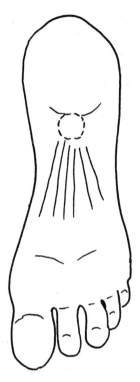

Figure 12.6   Site of tenderness in plantar fasciitis

Physical Treatment

Physiotherapy

This is not the place to review the whole range of physiotherapy treatments and their uses and abuses.

The doctor should get to know his or her local physiotherapy department and its strengths and weaknesses. The major areas of expertise that should be sought are assessment, physical treatment, especially exercise, and patient education. As a rule the 'prescription' card should ask for 'Assess and treat' rather than for specific therapy. Hence the therapist should be carefully choosing the best treatment, based on a constant re-assessment of the patient. However, the therapist must be prepared to justify the treatments chosen and should be able to provide a detailed assessment for the clinical notes. In most rheumatic conditions the most important treatment modality is exercise. The muscles are the best defence against joint damage. Most electrical treatments have yet to be shown to be effective in rheumatic diseases. Patient education is a major role for the therapist in the rheumatic diseases. This includes the important topics of joint protection and basic information about the disease process, to supplement what the doctor has been able to tell the patient.

Occupational therapy

In rheumatology the occupational therapist has several roles. These include assessment of daily living skills, the teaching of new ways of replacing lost skills, the provision of technical aids, assessment for wheelchairs, home visiting, liaison with Social Services and Housing Departments, and assisting the physiotherapist with exercise therapy by providing task-related activities that will improve patient motivation. The assessments that the occupational therapists provide form an important part of the clinical record.

Social intervention

The social worker has available a wide range of skills and resources to aid the rheumatic patient. These range from help with claiming appropriate financial benefits, applying to Housing Departments for home modifications or rehousing, contacting self-help groups, arranging home-helps, meals-on-wheels and holidays, and providing counselling for the patient and his or her relatives. It is important to remember that arthritis can be disabling not only in the physical sense but also psychologically. Every patient with chronic rheumatic disease should be made aware that a social worker is available and willing to help with any problems that arise.

Surgery

Readers are referred to orthopaedic texts for a full discussion of the role of surgery in the rheumatic conditions. A few general observations will be made here about the selection of suitable patients and the role of the physician in assisting the surgeon in pre- and postoperative care.

Surgery can be used in a variety of ways. It can be used:

1 to prevent joint damage – synovectomy;
2 reconstruction
    osteotomy
    tendon repair
    carpal tunnel release
    removal of prolapsed disc;

3   joint replacement
        hip
        knee
        ankle
        metacarpo-phalangeal joints;
4   salvage
        arthrodesis
        amputation

With complex joint problems, it is important to remember that replacing, say, the hip joint will not solve the patient's problem if there is still knee and ankle disease. It is also important to consider the reasons for undertaking surgery. Hence, with the hip there are a number of indications – night pain, difficulty walking, and problems with sexual intercourse. Knee surgery has to be done against the background of the complexities of the joint, which is not only a hinge between the femur and tibia but also has a rotational component to lock the knee in standing and the patellofemoral joint. Care must be taken to select the best type of prosthesis if replacement is to be considered, and the patient must be assessed for suitability for operation. This includes the general health and the willingness of the patient to undertake rehabilitation after the operation.

Prior to operation the full details should be discussed with the patient. Many rheumatoid patients will be anaemic and this may require transfusion if the anaesthetist and surgeon feel it appropriate. If the patient is on steroids it will be necessary to increase the dose over the period of the surgery. If possible the muscle groups around the joint to be operated on should be built up.

In the postoperative stage adequate analgesia should be offered. A careful watch must be kept on the haemoglobin. Mobilisation should be undertaken as soon as possible, using walking aids if necessary in lower-limb surgery. Considerable care must be taken to ensure that the wound remains clean, and infection should be treated promptly should it occur.

FURTHER READING

Ansell, B. M. (1980) *Rheumatic Disorders in Childhood*. London: Butterworths.

Benjamin, A. and Helal, B. (1980) *Surgical Repair and Reconstruction in Rheumatoid Disease*. London: Macmillan Publications.

Boyle, A. C. (1980) *A Colour Atlas of Rheumatology*, 2nd. edn. London: Wolfe Medical Publications Ltd.

Clarke, A. K. and Allard, L. L. (1986) *Rheumatology – the Team Approach to Rehabilitation*. London: Martin Dunitz.

Currey, H. L. F. (1980) *Mason and Currey's Clinical Rheumatology*, 3rd. edn. London, Pitman.

Dieppe, P. A., Bacon, P. A., Bamji, A. N. *et al.* (1982) *Slide Atlas of Rheumatology*. London: Gower Medical Publishing Ltd.

Dieppe, P. A., Doherty, M., McFarlane, D. G. and Maddison, P. J. (1985) *Rheumatological Medicine*. Edinburgh: Churchill Livingstone.

Dixon, A. St. J. and Graber, J. (1983) *Local Injection Therapy in Rheumatic Diseases*. Basle: Eular Publishers.

Golding, D. N. (1982) *A Synopsis of Rheumatic Diseases*, 4th edn. Bristol: Wright (John) & Sons Ltd.

Hart, F. D. (1983) *Practical Problems in Rheumatology*. London: Martin Dunitz.

Hughes, G. V. R. (1979) *Connective Tissue Diseases*, 2nd edn. Oxford, Blackwell Scientific Publications.

Huskisson, E. C. and Hart, F. D. (1978) *Joint Disease: all the arthropathies*. Bristol: Wright (John) & Sons Ltd.

Jayson, M. I. V. (1980) *The Lumbar Spine and Back Pain*, 2nd edn. London: Pitman.

Kelly, W. N., Harris, E. D., Ruddy, S. *et al.* (1981) *Textbook of Rheumatology*. Philadelphia: Saunders (W.B.) Co. Inc.

McCarty, D. J. (1979) *Arthritis and Allied Conditions*, 9th edn. Philadelphia: Lea & Febiger.

Moll, J. M. H. (1980) *Ankylosing Spondylitis*. Edinburgh: Churchill Livingstone.

Riggs, G. K. and Gall, E. P. (1981) *Rheumatic Diseases: rehabilitation and management*. Boston: Butterworths.

Rodnan, G. P. and Schumacher, H. R. (1983) *Primer on the Rheumatic Diseases*, 8th edn. Atlanta: Arthritis Foundation.

Wright, V. (ed.) (1982) *Topical Reviews in Rheumatic Diseases*, vol. 2. Bristol: Wright (John) & Sons Ltd.

Wynn Parry, C. B. (1981) *Rehabilitation of the Hand*, 4th edn. London: Butterworths.

INDEX

233